PSYCHIATRY IN MEDICINE

A SYMPOSIUM HELD AT
THE SCHOOL OF MEDICINE
UNIVERSITY OF CALIFORNIA,
LOS ANGELES
MARCH 10-11, 1961
TO MARK THE OPENING OF
THE NEUROPSYCHIATRIC INSTITUTE

Symposium on Psychiatry in Medicine, University of California at Los Angeles, 1961

PSYCHIATRY

IN

MEDICINE; [papers]

EDITED BY NORMAN Q. BRILL, M.D.

UNIVERSITY OF CALIFORNIA PRESS

BERKELEY AND LOS ANGELES, 1962

University of California Press

Berkeley and Los Angeles, California

Cambridge University Press

London, England

© 1962 by The Regents of the University of California

Library of Congress Catalog Card Number: 62-11489

Designed by Frank J. Lieberman

Printed in the United States of America

PREFACE

A SYMPOSIUM on Psychiatry in Medicine was held at the UCLA School of Medicine on March 10 and 11, 1961, to mark the opening of the Neuropsychiatric Institute. A guiding principle in the planning of the institute was the importance of closely integrating its structure and operation with the rest of the Medical Center.

Although emotional problems are encountered in medical practice more often than any other type of disorder, this aspect of medical education has been relatively neglected. The average medical school graduate is quite capable of treating most organic diseases, but he is usually not adequately prepared to diagnose and to treat emotional and functional disorders, nor does he understand sufficiently the important role that emotion plays in many organic disorders.

In part, this failure has stemmed from the isolation of psychiatric treatment facilities from the rest of medical treatment facilities, and this has impaired the proper integrating of psychiatric teaching with the rest of medical training. When psychiatric facilities are set apart, even by a small distance, from those of other medical disciplines, there is danger that student and patient alike will look upon the treatment of emotional illness as something apart from medicine.

Psychiatric treatment has changed radically in the past fifteen years, with a shift away from commitment and custodial care in isolated hospitals toward early active treatment in the general hospital. There has been a significant increase in the understanding of the intimate relation between psyche and soma. It has become increasingly clear that the responsibility for dealing with the many manifestations of emotional problems belongs to all physicians and particularly to the general practitioner.

The Department of Psychiatry has for several years been coöperating with the Division of Continuing Education in Medicine of the UCLA Extension in the postgraduate training of general practitioners. Generous support from the U.S. Public Health Service, National Institute of Mental Health, has made this program possible. The symposium on Psychiatry in Medicine was part of this program. It was designed for physicians who wished to attain greater understanding of the emotional disorders encountered in practice and greater effectiveness in the treatment of such disorders.

The topics covered in the series of lectures presented at the symposium were selected to achieve (in part) this purpose. The intricacies of the dynamics of psychophysiological reactions are reviewed by Dr. Felix Deutsch. By examples drawn from experimental work with animals and human subjects, he describes the role of unconscious forces in the production of physical disorders. The roots of psychosomatic disorders are seen as originating early in life when psycho-biological reaction patterns become established. These patterns are often unobserved and escape clinical detection. They are later found to be motivated by appropriate stimuli. A disturbing idea in being repressed may become attached to some part of the body and thereby affect its function. Using classical psychoanalytical formulations, Dr. Deutsch explains somatization as a transformation of libido by innate mechanisms which are designed to maintain psychic equilibrium. He raises the hope that further knowledge of the reticular activating system may provide the long-sought biological foundation for bridging the gap between mind and body.

In a presentation by Dr. Eric D. Wittkower, psychological problems of sick patients and of the doctors who treat them are outlined. Existing or approaching illness may manifest itself by withdrawal of interest from the environment. Using the defense mechanism of denial, a patient may attribute his malaise to trivial causes, and later develop exaggerated anxiety when this mechanism begins to fail as a result of the mounting stimuli from the progressing disease. The point is made that minor degrees of anxiety in response to a diagnosis may be desirable for the acceptance of the sick role. If infantile fantasies in the doctor have not been adequately curbed by reality testing, the doctor may be pompous and conceited, and blind to his own limitations, and he may thus be tempted to undertake professional tasks for which he is not qualified. There is always the danger that he may not recognize the regressive dependent motives behind his patients' fantasies, and may use them to feed his own self-adulation.

Preface

Dr. George L. Engel advances the argument that what is humanistic in medicine has also a scientific basis. He maintains that, when the concept of disease is sufficiently broadened to permit consideration of all the determinants (physical, chemical, biological, genetic, morphologic, psychologic, interpersonal, and social), the therapeutic significance of the personal and social aspects of medical care becomes more understandable. He examines some of the early determinants in terms of object relationships and self-concepts, and considers the evidence in both humans and animals that disruption of the valued object relationships constitutes a psychological stress which, under certain conditions, may eventuate in disease. Conversely, dynamic processes operating in the framework of the doctor-patient relationship and medical care may have restitutive or therapeutic value.

Some ecological and spiritual factors that are involved in human adaption are explored by Dr. Stewart Wolf. He believes the very fact that the evolution of man's behavior has outrun the evolution of his bodily form and functionings may be pertinent to maladaptations and to development of disease. He reminds us that there was a time when man's conception of society was more primitive, when the appropriate way to deal with an opponent was to kill and eat him. At that time, perhaps, the linking of gastric hypersecretion of acid and pepsin with circumstances that aroused hostility and resentment may have been an appropriate adaptation gradually established over millions of years. During the past several thousand years, however, man's conception of society has been changing from a primary emphasis on competition to a greater concern with interdependence and coöperative living. More recently we have been moving in the direction of considering that man should be his brother's keeper. The altered behavior that results from such altered attitudes "has left no enemy flesh in his [man's] stomach and nothing for his digestive juices to work on but his civilized meals and his own tissues." He suggests that now the need is for man to modulate his emotional as well as his behavioral responses to people. Perhaps he needs to "love his enemy and hate him not."

The need to respect the protective nature of mental illness is emphasized by Dr. Douglas D. Bond, who is concerned with the human approach to medicine and who establishes a valid foundation for the art of medicine through vignettes of his patients.

In reviewing the broad subject of children's emotional problems, Dr. George E. Gardner recognizes that certain stresses and crises occur in the life of every child at various age levels, merely because he is a human being living among other human beings and in a society, both personal and material, which generates threats of danger. This is natural because of the inherent vulnerability of the child to the effects of his smallness and his weakness. The solution of problems at each stage of development in large part determines his success or failure in tasks inevitably presented to the child as he grows older. There is an "optimal emotional climate" that should surround the child if he is to learn to solve problems successfully—a climate in which love, attention, warmth, and acceptance are expressed and enjoyed by all the persons (and particularly by the mother) surrounding the child in babyhood and early life. This climate alone and the sense of security it generates within the child will enable him to withstand the frustrations, delays, and denials (to the continuation of the full and unmodified expression of his instinctual drives) which are not only inevitably the lot of the infant and the child but essential if the child is to develop.

In dealing with problems at the other end of life's span —the emotional problems of aging—Dr. Maurice E. Linden cautions against the marked tendency to regard the problems of oldsters merely as the problems of youngsters grown old. This notion may be the basis of the mistaken belief that any therapist or practitioner who possesses skill in the management of the emotional problems of any other age group must, perforce, be competent to deal with older people. Effective treatment for an older person must be based on an understanding that he is a product of his culture, a member of a sociologic group. He is the culmination of a massive aggregate of intrapsychic phenomena, and hence an individual with specific neurotic needs which arose in childhood, were influenced by living, and were exaggerated by the stresses of aging.

The cultural rejection of the elderly person has created a special group of problems with their accompanying psychopathological reactions. Elderly people are not afforded status and privilege in our culture, which is primarily child-centered and youth-oriented. Instead of enjoying a feeling of dignity, they are made to feel superfluous. Social mobility, materialism, and overevaluation of sexuality and physical attractiveness leave the older person feeling rejected, or even excluded. His conservatism contributes to his feeling of (and, at times, actual) isolation from the rapidly changing culture. There is a tendency to react with depression, which is often disguised by other symptoms.

Dr. Karl Menninger describes the change that has taken place in the concept of diagnosis as the intellectual world has moved from static to dynamic ways of perceiving experience. "With the advance of medical knowledge the whole ontologic notion of disease as the invasion of the body by a foreign body no longer correctly represents medical thinking. The recognition of disease as an aspect of human existence, a phase of altered conditions of functioning in the life history of an individual interacting with an environment, requires us to abandon old names and old diagnostic methods. Treatment is, after all, the basic medical function, and diagnosis must serve the needs and purposes of treatment. Hence it must supply an accurate analysis of the illness processes so as to guide the physician in rational efforts toward an effective intervention."

Mr. Albert Deutsch, who spent several years surveying current psychiatric research in America, speaks of its explosive expansion in recent years and of the improvement in its quality. He is impressed by the breadth, the intensity, and the variety of current research, and by the diversity of scientists engaged in it. In view of the great public interest in announcements of new treatments, he warns against overenthusiastic claims which lead to sensational stories of "miracle cures," such as those that occurred with the introduction of tranquilizing drugs. Mr. Deutsch points out that such stories, although tending to enliven public interest and stimulate public support of psychiatric research, carry with them the danger inherent in repeated disillusionment—a resigned and cynical public apathy. It seems to him that there is too much talk of breakthroughs on the therapeutic front, even among psychiatrists. "This exaggeration of research accomplishments gives the false impression that the big one-shot cure for mental disease is just around the corner. The public must be made more aware of the very great problems that await solution. It must be better informed of the years and years of painstaking basic research behind such spectacular developments as the atomic bomb, the Salk vaccine, and most new therapies that burst seemingly full-blown before the public eye."

As an introduction to the symposium, I attempted to reappraise the psychotherapeutic process.

The symposium was planned and conducted by Drs. Frank F. Tallman, Charles W. Tidd, Charles W. Wahl, Ivan N. Mensh, Edward J. Kollar, and Henry H. Work, all of the UCLA Department of Psychiatry. I am indebted to them for their generous help, and to my secretary, Mrs. Margaret Conover, for all her assistance in making arrangements and in typing manuscripts. To Miss Betty Minifie and her staff in the office of Continuing Education in Medicine of University Extension go our special thanks for their many efforts in making the symposium possible. We are particularly grateful to the UCLA Medical Center Auxiliary and to a pharmaceutical firm, which has contributed actively to the support of psychiatric education and research, for their generosity which enabled us to publish this volume.

Norman Q. Brill, M.D.

CONTRIBUTORS

NORMAN Q. BRILL, M.D.

Professor of Psychiatry, University of California, Los Angeles

KARL MENNINGER, M.D., D.SC.

Director of Education and Dean of Menninger School of Psychiatry, Menninger Foundation; Chief of Staff, Menninger Clinic; Clinical Professor of Psychiatry, University of Kansas School of Medicine

GEORGE L. ENGEL, M.D.

Professor of Psychiatry and Associate Professor of Medicine, University of Rochester School of Medicine

DOUGLAS D. BOND, M.D.

Professor of Psychiatry and Dean, Western Reserve

Contributors

School of Medicine, University Hospitals, Cleveland, Ohio

STEWART G. WOLF, JR., M.D.

Professor and Chairman, Department of Medicine, Consultant Professor of Psychiatry and Neurology, University of Oklahoma Medical Center

FELIX DEUTSCH, M.D.

Honorary Professor of Psychiatry, Boston University; Senior Training Analyst, Boston Psychoanalytic Institute

MAURICE E. LINDEN, M.D.

Director, Division of Mental Health, Department of Public Health, Philadelphia; Assistant Professor of Psychiatry, University of Pennsylvania School of Medicine

ALBERT DEUTSCH

Author and Lecturer

ERIC D. WITTKOWER, M.D.

Associate Professor of Psychiatry, McGill University and Allan Memorial Institute, Montreal

GEORGE E. GARDNER, PH.D., M.D.

Director, Judge Baker Guidance Center, Boston; Psychiatrist-in-Chief, Children's Hospital Medical Center, Boston; Clinical Professor of Psychiatry, Harvard Medical School

CONTENTS

Contents

1 THE PSYCHO-

THERAPEUTIC PROCESS

BY NORMAN Q. BRILL, M.D.

I WOULD LIKE to explain why Psychiatry in Medicine was chosen as the theme for this symposium. It would be difficult to conceive of a symposium entitled Pediatrics in Medicine or Obstetrics in Medicine, but psychiatry as a specialty seems to occupy a somewhat different position from other specialties. It deals with disturbed people rather than with disturbed organs or organ systems. The practice of other specialties is based much more on the sciences of anatomy, pathology, physiology, pharmacology, and physiological chemistry than is the practice of psychiatry, which is based much more (but by no means exclusively) on the science of psychology and, increasingly, on sociology and cultural anthropology.

For many years psychiatry used institutions and sanitariums, while other specialties used hospitals. Psychiatry provided custody; hospitals provided treatment. Psychiatry's concepts and language were different. Psychopathology was described as disturbances in thinking, feeling, and acting, and not in terms of the more familiar cellular infiltrations, vascular lesions, or degenerative changes.

Judging from a resolution passed by the American Psychiatric Association ninety years ago, even a description of the various types of psychoses was not routinely taught in medical schools. Four conferences on psychiatric education, held in the years 1933–1936 under the auspices of the National Committee for Mental Hygiene, and a survey of psychiatry in medical education by Drs. Ebaugh and Rymer (8), published in 1942, emphasized the inadequacies of psychiatric teaching at that time. The Ithaca Conference on Psychiatric Education, held in 1951, once again attempted to improve psychiatric education in medical schools. It emphasized, among other things, the need for instruction in personality development, psychodynamics, and interviewing, a far cry from the purely descriptive psychiatry of the last century.

Along with changes in medical education came changes in the treatment of psychiatric patients. Institutions became hospitals; treatment was emphasized rather than custody. Today we find that psychiatric hospitals are playing an active role in training and in research and that there is an increasing trend away from commitment to voluntary treatment in general hospitals.

The awareness of the role emotions play in producing somatic disease is vastly increased. Study of the difficult, uncoöperative, and depressed patient has highlighted the importance of emotional factors in the treatment of patients with organic disease. The frequency with which physicians are consulted by patients with symptoms of primarily emotional origin is more clearly recognized.

The Psychotherapeutic Process

Medication alone is not sufficient to relieve many of the cases of peptic ulcer, ulcerative colitis, anorexia nervosa, asthma, and dermatitis which the physician is called upon to treat. Insulin is of little value for the diabetic who refuses to take it, and diet does not help the obese patient who neglects or is unable to follow it. Operations do not cure the surgical addict, and hearing aids do not assist the person who does not want to hear.

Recognition of this has made it important to develop a closer integration of psychiatry with medicine. It has become essential for all doctors to study the science of psychiatry and to learn about the nature and the implications of the doctor-patient relationship, and about the techniques of psychotherapy which are intimately connected with this relationship.

The vital role of the physician in any mental health program has been emphasized by Dr. E. V. Askey, president of the American Medical Association. He points out that "the general practitioner or the specialist in some field other than psychiatry often has a greater opportunity to help his patients maintain their mental health than does the psychiatrist. He must seize that opportunity and use it to its fullest. He can do so only if he is armed with an adequate body of psychiatric knowledge and the disposition to use it. Given these he can be astonishingly effective in early diagnosis of mental illness and in the treatment of some forms of mental disease." He does not suggest that the practice of psychiatry be turned over to the general practitioner, but he does insist that "every doctor can and must become an effective practitioner of total medicine—for the physician who practices total medicine contributes massively to preventive measures, helps make treatment available more quickly and helps establish mental health more solidly as a concept vital to every community. One thing is certain: The psychiatrist alone cannot do the job that needs to be done. He is spread too thin as it is. He needs the help and cooperation of doctors in every type of practice" (4).

The need for this development is acute because there are many other individuals who would like, for a variety of reasons not always concerned with interest in the patient, to take over this responsibility. If the medical profession does not assume it, these others will, and what progress has been made over a span of many years is getting "psyche" and "soma" together may then be lost.

Doctors, often without being aware of it, tend to feel contempt for patients with emotional disorders. A survey of medical students' attitudes toward patients, by Geertsma, Mac-Andrew, and Stoller (11), reveals that the kind of patient doctors like the least has the characteristics of the psychiatric patient. It would seem to be the duty of a medical faculty to alter these attitudes in their students. One way of doing this is to give the same priority and emphasis to the diagnosis and the treatment of emotional disorders, regardless of their manifestation, as is given to other forms of illness. This is done in part by providing psychiatric facilities along with all others in a teaching hospital. It is this purpose that prompted the construction of the Neuropsychiatric Institute as an integral part of the Medical Center at the University of California, Los Angeles. Psychiatry will not be something set apart from the rest of the hospital. Perhaps in time the stigma that still exists for emotional illnesses will disappear; perhaps in the future patients and their families will not wait so long before seeking help.

The interrelationship between psychiatry and medicine is so intimate that any separation of the two will be deterimental to the advance of both. That mental illness is in some way associated with brain dysfunction is now widely accepted. The nature of the dysfunction may vary from gross structural disorders in the brain (such as brain tumors; brain infections; deficiency states; posttraumatic lesions; and metabolic, genetic, and circulatory disturbances) to more subtle disturbances in function such as are now being revealed by modern physiological and biochemical techniques of investigation.

There is much to suggest that schizophrenia is a psychosomatic disorder in which brain function is impaired as a consequence of, or an accompaniment to, emotional conflict. The symptoms of schizophrenia clearly indicate that the brain is not functioning properly. The impairment of thinking, feeling, and acting in the schizophrenic would appear to be related to brain dysfunction as much as vomiting is related to stomach dysfunction of psychic or emotional origin.

The impaired reactivity of chronic regressed schizophrenics to stimlui and to drugs of various kinds is additional evidence of some dysfunction of the central nervous system. I do not mean to suggest that there is a space-occupying lesion or one that can be demonstrated by present histological techniques, but a disturbance must be present in the physiology or the chemistry of the cells, or there must be interference with the interaction between groups of cells. The prolonged autistic withdrawal of the chronic schizophrenic who has turned his attention away from the world of reality may cause him to lose the ability to perceive reality in the way that an unused strabismic eye eventually loses its ability to see.

Hernandez-Peon (16) has shown in experiments on animals how the amplitude of electrical responses evoked in the brain by auditory stimuli decrease as the animal loses interest in the stimuli. His findings suggest that the response of the cochlear nucleus of a cat is dependent upon excitation from higher centers and that a stimulus that has presumably ceased to have any meaning or importance to the cat hardly even registers in the brain. Arieti (3) has postulated some such disturbance in functional integration of the brain in schizophrenia, and believes that irreversible changes occur in the brains of regressed patients who have been sick for a long time. It is likely that neurophysiological disturbances will be convincingly demonstrated before long. Heath (14), Sem-Jacobsen (22), and others have already reported suggestive findings, but they still await confirmation.

Recent advances in drug therapy have stimulated a great dependence on pharmacological methods of approach. New techniques in microhistology and the electron microscope promise to make important contributions to the understanding of mental illness.

The mental health of a person is so intimately linked to his physical health that good psychiatric practice must be superimposed upon and dependent on good medical practice. This can be achieved only through the continued integration of psychiatric instruction with other departments in medical schools—at both the undergraduate and the graduate levels.

There has been an implication that medicine's approach to psychiatry must change. Admittedly many changes are needed in psychiatry also. The psychiatric consultant is often criticized for confirming the existence of an emotional disorder and then not doing anything about it except to recommend psychotherapy. Have we failed to convince our medical colleagues that psychotherapy is effective? Do they refuse to recognize instances when it has been helpful, or have we failed to demonstrate sufficiently that it can be helpful?

M. Kaufman (18) challenges anything but an extremely eclectic role for the psychiatrist who, he feels, has to relate himself to every aspect of the practice of medicine. He states that

> *one of the basic facts of life in regard to a psychiatrist in a general hospital is the simple and pragmatic one as to whether he is of any value to the other members of the staff. The surgeon or the internist is not interested, except in an academic way, as to what the diagnostic label is or in what to him very frequently is an esoteric evaluation of psychodynamic factors for their own sake. He is, however, interested as a physician and as a practitioner of medicine in a colleague's help to understand and to be of practical assistance in the total evaluation and furtherance of treatment of any given patient. He does not sell a psychiatric point of view if he disguises himself with a false face and pretends to erudition that is essentially superficial.*

Have we confused our colleagues by speaking of psychotherapy without defining it, as one might recommend medication without saying what kind, what dose, and to what end?

There are many different kinds of psychotherapy, many possible techniques and goals, and there must be some indication for the selected form in each case. Has this been emphasized sufficiently? Do some of us plunge into psychotherapy without our knowing (or the patient's knowing) where we are going, how long it will take, and the result to be expected? Is more confusion created when at times we encourage, sanction, or tolerate psychiatric treatment by persons of widely varying backgrounds and training, whose only justification is interest instead of competence?

What kind of treatment is psychotherapy if it must not be interrupted by a phone call to the doctor, or a knock on the door, except in an emergency? What kind of treatment is it if it is presumed to start with the first interview before a diagnosis is established and a goal of treatment decided upon? I do not mean to suggest that these questions apply to all psychiatrists, or even to the majority of them, but we must admit that there is a realistic basis for inquiring.

To be sure, the tone for the treatment process may be set by the first interview, and the mere going to a psychiatrist for help may have a significant psychotherapeutic effect. How the first interview is conducted may have a great and continuing influence on the subsequent course of treatment, but this does not mean that the first exploratory interview actually is treatment. We need to define more exactly the contraindications, if any, and the special indications for psychotherapy, as well as the qualifications and the training of the physician (or of anyone else) who assumes the responsibility for such treatment.

Psychotherapy may be broadly defined as the systematized, goal-directed use of psychological measures, or other measures having a psychological effect, for the treatment of mental and emotional disorders. It must be differentiated from the psychotherapeutic effect which may accompany many procedures, anticipated or not. I would no more consider a housewife's comforting of a neighbor as psychotherapy than I would consider as practicing medicine her suggestion that a friend take an aspirin for a headache. The doctor who informs a worried patient that her physical examination is negative, and thereby relieves her anxiety, is not necessarily doing psychotherapy.

Many variables will influence the type of psychotherapy to be undertaken: the nature of the patient's illness; the patient's age, sex, and financial status; the patient's motivation, psychological-mindedness, cultural background, intelligence, ego strength, and desire to change; the availability of treatment resources, the presence or absence of coexisting organic disease; external precipitating factors; and the competence and the interest of the psychiatrist. The kind of treatment will be determined also by the goal selected. It may be to help the patient become happier, to relieve symptoms, to increase his frustration tolerance, to help him better understand himself and his illness, or to produce a change in his personality and character structure.

Unfortunately there has been a widespread tendency to equate psychotherapy and psychoanalysis. Psychiatric literature is replete with examples of authors who use the two terms interchangeably. This further confuses the issue and, because of the higher status that psychoanalysis presently enjoys in the United States, some psychiatrists employ psychoanalytic techniques and interpretations and half believe they are "doing psychoanalysis."

It is frequently said that only those who want to be helped can be helped; that the alcoholic who is wrecking his own and his family's life cannot be helped unless he wants help and seeks it. It is unfortunate that the lack of motivation to seek help is not in itself regularly and constantly looked upon as a symptom that is masochistic or self-destructive. Admittedly, such a symptom is often extremely difficult to control, but this should serve as an incentive for the development of more adequate methods of dealing with it. Very often children can be motivated to coöperate in treatment even though they do not themselves actively seek help. Perhaps the same thing is true of many adults.

Unfortunately, because more people actively seek treatment than can be taken care of, the person with negative motivation is likely to be pushed aside. It is said that he will have to get worse and suffer more before he can get better. His lack of control is not always recognized, and the physician too often unknowingly joins the patient's family in hostile, impotent procrastination and passivity, or outright rejection.

Society will tolerate and ignore the skid-row alcoholic who is slowly destroying himself, whereas it would not ignore a person obviously bleeding to death. Some skid-row alcoholics punish themselves in the hope that an "angel of mercy" will see how they are suffering and come to help them. They may refuse the help when it is offered while secretly yearning for it, and needing it, to overcome their martyrdom.

Psychiatrists, and particularly psychiatrists in training, often believe they help the patient by *what* they do, that is, by uncovering dynamics, which may be considered a "scientific" approach, rather than by *how* they do it. Taking an interest in the patient, being sympathetic and understanding, hopeful and reassuring, seems more like the witch doctor, shaman, or priest method, which is less scientific and therefore less valuable. But having positive feelings toward a patient, though at times a detriment, is not always undesirable. It can often be helpful.

In psychoanalysis, the feelings of the analyst toward the patient may stem from the analyst's endowing the patient with attitudes and characteristics of persons important in his early life. Such feelings will interfere with the analyst's objectivity and true understanding of the patient. It is therefore important to identify such countertransference feelings and eliminate them.

It is not uncommon to find this principle extended to psychotherapy and accompanied by the belief that, if the therapist's conscious and unconscious feelings toward the patient are eliminated, the patient's problem will be clarified. This would presuppose that everyone has the same astuteness, sensitivity, logic, adroitness, and skill to mobilize when emotional involvement with the patient is resolved through personal analysis or individual determination. It also presupposes that all therapists are equally emancipated, so that any one of them, regardless of the duration and the nature of his clinical experience, is capable of great insight. It is important to realize that it is not always personal difficulties that prevent the doctor from understanding the meaning of what the patient says or does, as has been pointed out by R. Waelder (25).

Because many doctors possess enough sensitivity and

understanding to help patients with emotional problems, all physicians are somehow expected to be capable of doing psychotherapy after relatively little training in medical school and in internship. It would appear, from the frequency with which beginning psychiatric residents are encouraged to assume responsibilities far beyond their experience and competence, that even the residents and often their teachers do not realize that training is necessary.

It is believed by some that the effectiveness of psychotherapy is often more related to the therapist's investment and confidence in his particular technique (and in the theoretical framework underlying it) and to the patient's investment in the therapist than it is to the technique itself.[1] Who uses the technique and how the patient feels about him become important factors in determining the outcome of the therapy—perhaps at times more important than the technique itself. The effectiveness of drugs has been shown to be intimately related to the confidence in them which is conveyed by the physician to the patient, and the dramatic effect of placebos is similarly explained.

Most physicians who seek psychiatric training are primarily interested in learning how to do psychotherapy, as surgical residents are interested in learning how to do surgery. The surgeon is often suspected of recommending surgery for a particular condition primarily because of his skill. An internist, seeing the same patient, might recommend a more conservative medical treatment. One may presume

[1] M. Balint has pointed out that it is necessary for a teacher of psychotherapy to have conviction about the method if he is to be effective.

that the psychotherapeutically trained psychiatrist may likewise be suspected of recommending his particular ware when it may not be so clearly or specifically indicated as he thinks.

Psychiatrists often predict dire consequences for a patient who refuses psychotherapy, and yet there are many instances in which such consequences do not materialize. This may be the result of chance or of inability to predict failure, as described by Glass (12), but it seems likely that in some instances the psychiatrist's sense of urgency is a by-product of his own bias. Board found that even patients who were considered therapeutic failures reported improvement on follow-up (5). This is probably true of difficult patients who feel that the doctor is interested in them.

The student of surgery has the advantage of being able (and required) to watch his teacher, to have each step of the technique explained as it is performed, and eventually to imitate. The surgeon-teacher presumably knows why he is doing what he does. He ties off blood vessels or excises diseased tissue for straightforward reasons.

Until recently, students of psychotherapy have not had the same opportunity to observe their teachers and, more importantly, most teachers have been resistive, if not openly opposed, to being observed in the process of treating a patient, especially a private patient. To some extent this has been because observation might possibly have an ill effect on the patient, and especially on his ability freely to verbalize his thoughts and feelings. Though these considerations appear to have validity, the extent of the interference has not been determined by systematic investigation.

Perhaps of greater importance is the therapist's own

self-consciousness and his own reluctance to being observed. Intruders are usually no more welcome than they would be in the privacy of a bedroom. The therapist may not, like the surgeon, always be able to give a rational explanation for everything he did or said (i.e., rational in the sense that it was realistically indicated). Many times his speech or his actions may arise from his own thoughts, feelings, or impulses. In such instances the therapist would not be aware of the origins of his decisions and, if asked, would attempt to provide a seemingly rational explanation by pointing to something in the patient.

If the therapist, taking a cue from the psychoanalyst, maintains a neutral objective position in an attempt to avoid personal investment in, or emotional entanglement with, the patient, or gratification from any improvement the patient might show, he could still derive some gratification from the process itself. This may account in part for the marked appeal that the role of therapist has for psychologists, social workers, ministers, marriage counselors, teachers, nurses, and others.

There is probably more than ego satisfaction; there may be personal and subtle libidinal factors, and the extent of their involvement may be proportional to the reluctance of the therapist to be observed. It is as if something sexual were being exchanged between the patient and the therapist. This would account (at least in part) for the desire for complete privacy.

In places where the use of one-way mirrors was introduced for observing therapy, the therapist was far more uncomfortable than the patient when both knew they were being observed. The patient's attention is apt to be focused on the doctor, and the doctor's attention is apt to be divided between the patient and his unseen audience. The reluctance to be observed may stem not merely from conscious and unconscious concern about the personal performance, but indeed from lack of experience and lack of confidence. One who does not know what he is doing is not willing to be watched doing it.

The fear of giving a physical examination to a patient to be treated psychotherapeutically has been observed in both psychiatric residents and their faculty supervisors. The origin of this fear, which is more than simply reluctance, seems to be in part the rather wholesale application of psychoanalytic techniques to psychotherapy. The common rationalization is that the physical examination may provoke sexual fantasies in the patient or the patient may, through the examination, gratify sexual feelings or resist the psychotherapeutic process. The failure to deal with this resistance suggests, according to some psychiatrists, that the therapist derives sexual gratification from giving the physical examination or that his sexual wishes toward the patient are stimulated and interfere with his objectivity. Why can this difficulty not be uncovered and dealt with in consultation, as are other interfering feelings when they arise? [2]

According to Reusch (21), "Psychotherapy is less

[2] There are situations, of course, where a physical examination should be avoided if possible. Sometimes a paranoid patient has reacted to the physical examination as a sexual assault, or a homosexual patient has been thrown into panic or psychosis by a rectal examination. After many years of not doing physical examinations, psychiatrists may realistically have no confidence in their ability to elicit abnormal findings.

of a method and more of an experience and therapists make it possible for the patients to have such an experience; and experience, a truly private phenomenon, is not accessible to objective verification."

Liking a patient is ordinarily held to be the psychotherapist's prime prerequisite for treating a patient. Branch (6) states: "It may be stretching the matter too far to say that beginning residents should have in psychotherapy only patients they like." He quotes Knight (19), who says that "optimism and liking for the patient often go hand-in-hand as do pessimism and dislike for the patient . . . and he responds accordingly."

What does liking consist of? Judging from the choice of patients by residents, when given the chance, sexual elements appear to be quite prominent. They seem to select the youngest and the prettiest women. This may not be bad, for precisely this element of interest may be a critical factor in treatment. This does not mean that patients for whom there is no initial interest or libidinal investment cannot be helped, for of course interest may develop. Even in psychoanalysis—or, perhaps, especially in psychoanalysis—where interest interferes if it becomes personalized, the existence of interest of some kind permits the process, difficult for analyst and patient alike, to proceed.

The word "interest" means "mental excitement accompanying special attention to some object which may be intellectual, sympathetic, and emotional, or merely personal." One may, as an analyst, ignore the interest or render it innocuous by complete concentration on the meaning of a patient's productions, actions, and reactions, but the interest is still there and will reveal its existence to the patient. The importance of this to the entire psychotherapeutic or psychoanalytic process has never been accurately determined, although interest on the part of the therapist might be expected to be, for the psychiatric patient who almost universally feels involved, a *sine qua non*.

Heine (15) has emphasized the importance to patients of the personal characteristics of the therapist rather than of his technique. Perhaps this is a partial answer for Branch and Ely (7), who found it difficult to explain the enthusiasm for and popularity of psychotherapy, in the absence of valid statistical evidence of the effectiveness of psychotherapy derived from the comparison of treated and untreated groups.

Frank (9) found that psychiatric outpatients with psychoneurotic and personality disorders experienced similar subjective improvement, primarily a decrease in anxiety and depression, whether they were given individual therapy once a week, group therapy one and a half hours a week, or symptomatic treatment involving visits of no more than half an hour every two weeks. In fact, at the end of six months the patients who had dropped out of treatment within the first month showed the same incidence of subjective improvement as those who had remained in treatment for the six-month period.

It seemed to Frank that the relief of the patient's distress is related to the expectancy of help; that the effect is manifested very quickly and that its intensity is unrelated to the type and the duration of treatment; that the expectancy of help enables the patient to mobilize latent assets, creates a more favorable condition for learning, and contributes to more effective functioning; and that the improvement may be quite persistent and lasting. In some of his patients it lasted for two years even without a continuing contact with a therapist. Frank believed that the failure of studies to reveal any over-all difference in improvement rates of different therapies (e.g., the report of Appel [2]) may be due to the factor of "improvement from expectancy of help," a common factor in all therapies.

Frank (10) believes that even when the therapist tries not to influence the patient directly, mere prolonged contact of the patient with someone who has faith in his particular method of therapy will result in the patient's internalizing the values and the attitude of the therapist.

Hill (17) emphasizes that "being" and "doing" in therapy cannot be separated. "A therapist is what he does," and what he does is an expression of what he is. "The choice of what to do, what patients to treat, what goals to set, what techniques to use, or the choice from moment to moment whether to say something or not, or to do something or not; the choice of strategy for the long pull or the tactic of the moment is a choice which is made by the therapist as a predetermined expression of what he is, both as a person and as a therapist." What he is and what his interest in the patient is will necessarily be revealed to the patient and will determine, at least in part, the patient's response.

Franz Alexander (1) has also been impressed by the importance of the therapist as a variable. He states: "It is becoming clear to us that the influences of the *individuality of the therapist* is a crucial, although yet almost completely unexplored factor." Although appearing to equate analysis and therapy, Alexander raises very pertinent questions.

> *A further crucial question is how much, apart from his specific countertransference reactions, the therapist as a distinct individual enters into the therapeutic process. Or, in other words, would the course of the treatment be the same if the patient were treated by a different* analyst *with the same theoretical orientation and practical experience, but having a different personality; for example, had the patient been treated by a woman instead of by a man, by a younger man instead of an older man, by a reserved, rather than an outgoing personality—how are the specific personality features of the analyst, including his own value system, perceived by the patient even if the therapist tries to keep his incognito, and how does all this influence, if at all, the transference and the whole course of the treatment?*
>
> *These and many other vital questions are today unanswered. What seems to be certain is that the patient does not perceive the analyst only as an abstract intellect, but as a distinct person. This fact must be included in an adequate theory of the therapeutic process.*
>
> *It also appears to be certain that the emotional and the cognitive factors (in therapy) are organically connected. This fundamental fact makes the efforts to divide psychotherapeutic procedures, including psycho-*

analysis, into rigid categories, both artificial and futile. Knight [20] lucidly expressed this view in 1949, emphasizing that fundamentally there is only one psychotherapy which "must rest on a basic science of dynamic psychotherapy."

. . . Even emotional support alone may introduce spontaneous insight by decreasing anxiety which interferes with insight. In fact, I suspect that the supportive effect of the psychoanalytic process has not been sufficiently recognized as one of the main factors favoring both insight and the emergence of new emotional patterns.

. . . The emotional support which the patient derives from the treatment situation may restore the ego's temporarily impaired integrative capacity, and thus introduce a spontaneous healing process."

Strupp (23) suggests that psychotherapy is most effective when the therapist is able to relate to the patient in a warm, empathic manner so that the person of the therapist as revealed in this relationship will in time serve as a new, more mature, and more desirable model of reality than past interpersonal relationships which have distracted the patient's perceptions of himself and others. Interpretation and the other technical devices of therapy are least effective when this prime requisite is lacking.

Whitehorn has pointed out that what the therapist says to the patient has often been said previously by relatives and friends without effect. It is the relationship that exists, in reality or in fantasy between the patient and the therapist which lends force and meaning to the therapist's comments or interpretations. Symonds (24) observes that under quite different approaches a patient will use the therapeutic situation as his own need dictates, and that he will institute his own process of psychotherapy irrespective of the attitude the therapist takes toward him or the words that the therapist utters.

It has been repeatedly emphasized that the therapist, to be helpful, must have, as stated by Branch, "sufficient personal security to facilitate a helpful relationship to the patient and sufficient sophistication to promote adequate communication." Therapy must be used to assist the patient in functioning more effectively with his own assets and toward his own realistic goals, and not to satisfy the needs of the therapist.

The therapist approximates the understanding parent who is not trying to live his own life or to solve his own problems in the patient, or displacing attitudes and feelings upon the patient, but who is attempting, whatever the technique, to guide, advise, and help the patient to achieve constructive and realistic, and therefore happier, goals and to avoid the self-destructive, self-defeating tendencies that have brought him to treatment. To do this, the therapist must be able to deal with his own anxiety and to live with the concerns that a parent must necessarily tolerate in permitting a child to make mistakes and learn in the process of growing up.

The parent must, in the process of setting limits, be capable of enduring the anger and at times the hatred of the frustrated child without feeling obliged to strike back or get even. The therapist, too, must be capable of an enduring interest in the patient while being the object of transferred hate. The parents learn to accept the love of the child without succumbing to its attempted seductions (and without provoking them). So, too, the therapist must be capable of focusing on what is best for the patient by resisting the seductive efforts of the patient. Dr. Allen Wheelis (26) has shown how difficult this may be at times.

Increasing numbers of psychiatrists are spending years and making great financial and emotional sacrifices in order to obtain psychoanalytic training over and above the three years of residency required for American Board certification. The motivations are undoubtedly many, and the gratifications are equally numerous even if not obvious. Perhaps one important gratification in practicing psychoanalysis is like that of the parent who, by his own restraint, patience, and love, has guided his child through trying times to maturity. The gratifications, however, are not continually experienced. They are periodic and intermittent as each new stage is gone through and as advance becomes apparent. The therapist, like the parent, avoids bragging about his achievement but enjoys the rather controlled satisfaction of his accomplishment.

Haley (13) describes the patient's attempts to control the therapist, and concludes that the therapist must induce a patient voluntarily to behave differently from the way he has behaved in the past. The patient must imitate the new behavior and can be induced to do so only when direction on the part of the therapist is denied, giving the change in behavior the appearance of spontaneity. How like the methods parents must sometimes use with a difficult child! A prime example is the denial on the part of the parent of any sexual interest in the child, which aids the child in the resolution of his Oedipus complex and permits him to turn his interest elsewhere.

Perhaps in looking closely at the psychotherapeutic process we run the same danger as the proverbial centipede when he tried to discover how he coördinated his one hundred legs so beautifully: he lost the ability to walk. Interestingly, the observation has been made that some very successful psychotherapists lose their ability after personal psychoanalysis; they may become very competent psychoanalysts, but in the process they have learned to control or eliminate their own interaction with patients seeking and needing precisely this interaction. But there are many who, through better understanding of themselves, vastly improve their ability to treat the emotional problems of others.

References

1. ALEXANDER, F. Current problems in dynamic psychotherapy in its relationship to psychoanalysis. Am. J. Psychiat., 116:322–325, 1959.
2. APPEL, K. E., *et al.* Proceedings of the Assoc. for Research in Nervous and Mental Disease, 1951. Baltimore, Williams & Wilkins Co., 1953.
3. ARIETI, S. Interpretation of schizophrenia. New York, Robert Brunner, 1955.
4. ASKEY, E. V. Mental Hospitals, 12:18, 1961.
5. BOARD, F. A. Patients' and physicians' judgments of outcome of psychotherapy in an outpatient clinic. Arch. Gen. Psychiat., 1:185–196, 1959.
6. BRANCH, C. H., and J. W. ELY. Teaching the principles of ambulant psychotherapy. Am. J. Psychiat., 115:890, 1959.

7. *Ibid.,* p. 887.
8. EBAUGH, F. G., and C. A. RYMER. Psychiatry in medical education. New York, Commonwealth Fund, 1942.
9. FRANK, J. D., *et al.* Patients' expectancies and relearning as factors determining improvement in psychotherapy. Am. J. Psychiat., 115:961, 1959.
10. FRANK, J. D. The dynamics of the psychotherapeutic relationship. Psychiatry, 22:17–39, 1959.
11. GEERTSMA, R. H., C. MACANDREW, and R. J. STOLLER. Medical student orientations toward the emotionally ill. Arch. Neurol. & Psychiat., 81:377–383, 1959.
12. GLASS, A. J., *et al.* Psychiatric prediction and military effectiveness. U.S. Armed Forces Med. J., VII:1427–1442, 1955.
13. HALEY, J., JULES H. MASSERMAN, and J. L. MORENO. Progress in psychotherapy. New York, Grune & Stratton, 1959. Vol. IV, p. 65.
14. HEATH, R. G., *et al.* Studies in schizophrenia; a multidisciplinary approach to mind-brain relationships. Cambridge, Harvard University Press, 1954.
15. HEINE, R. W. A comparison of patients' reports on psychotherapeutic experience with psychoanalytic, nondirective and Adlerian therapists. Am. J. Psychotherapy, 7:16, 1953.
16. HERNANDEZ-PEON, R., and H. SCHERRER. "Habituation" to acoustic stimuli in cochlear nucleus. Federation Proc., 14:71, 1955.
17. HILL, L. B. On being rather than doing in psychotherapy. Intern. J. of Group Psychotherapy, VIII:115, 1958.
18. KAUFMAN, M. Use of the consultant: Workshop 1955. Orthopsych., 26:223–233, 1956.
19. KNIGHT, R. P. Psychotherapy of an adolescent catatonic schizophrenia with mutism. Psychiatry, 9:323, 1946.
20. KNIGHT, R. P. A critique of the present status of the psycho-

therapies. Bull. N.Y. Acad. Med., 2d series, 25 (no. 2):100–114, 1949.

21. REUSCH, J. Discussion of article by Branch and Ely. Am. J. Psychiat., 115:892, 1959.

22. SEM-JACOBSEN, C. W., *et al.* Electroencephalographic rhythms from the depths of the frontal lobe in 60 psychotic patients. EEG Clin. Neurophysiol., 7:193–210, 1955.

23. STRUPP, H. H. The psychotherapist's contribution to the treatment process. Behavioral Science, 3:34–67, 1958.

24. SYMONDS, P. M. Dynamics of psychotherapy. New York, Grune & Stratton, 1956. P. 13.

25. WAELDER, R., quoted by R. Ekstein. Report of a panel on the teaching of psychoanalytic technique (from the annual meeting of the Am. Psychoanalytic Assoc., April, 1959). J. Am. Psychoanal. Assoc., VIII (no. 1):169, 1960.

26. WHEELIS, A. The quest for identity. New York, W. W. Norton, 1958.

2 THE EVOLUTION

OF DIAGNOSIS*

BY KARL MENNINGER, M.D.

THE FIRST PART of our curriculum at the Menninger School of Psychiatry is devoted to intensive and extensive training in psychiatric case study in the examination of the psychiatric patient. Students often rebel at first at having to spend so much time in the study of diagnosis. They come with a strong inclination to treat someone who needs their merciful efforts. They recognize the theoretical place of diagnosis, but they are reluctant to apply themselves to the tedious details of acquiring the skills and the knowledge which modern psychiatric diagnosis requires.

Time was when a medical diagnosis could be made in one minute. A patient was asked to protrude his tongue, a hand was placed on his forehead and the doctor observed whether or not his face was flushed and asked about his bowels.

Something equivalent to this in psychiatric diagnosis sometimes occurs. I can recall when appointees of Massachusetts courts would come on a specified day of the week to the

* © 1961 by Karl Menninger.

Boston Psychopathic Hospital. They came in pairs and, pausing briefly before various patients in the wards, asked a few questions: Do you know what day it is? Do you hear voices? Does anyone have it in for you? Who is president of the United States? (I am sure a few of the questions were more sophisticated than these.) After a few minutes the "alienists" would pass on to another patient, and a few days later we received word that certain patients had been committed and would be duly transferred to Westboro or Danvers.

There are still colleagues who make psychiatric diagnoses in this way, but they bring our profession little credit. I do not think it is possible to make a psychiatric diagnosis, even for commitment purposes, in a few minutes or even in a few hours. I believe a psychiatric diagnosis should be based upon inquiries that take many hours, and our course in psychiatric case study endeavors to teach what should be done during these hours.

We go into much detail regarding psychiatric history-taking, emphasizing the differences between it and the medical case history. We indicate how many different histories have to be taken in every case in order to get a truly well-rounded picture of what various people think has happened or remember to have happened. We show, too, how the history, as we conclude it to have occurred, must be compared with the life history that the patient remembers or claims to remember, or, perhaps, does not remember.

Having concluded the history-taking, we proceed to the things that are taught in every good psychiatric clinic, I am sure, regarding examinations: the inspection, the investigation, and the description of the way the patient is discovered to be *right now*. This present state of existence is to be determined by the physical examination, combined with the neurological examination and with the data of the X-ray and the microscope and the test tube and all those paraphernalia of the chemical laboratory which have come to be a part of modern physical diagnosis. Finally, there is the psychological examination—the investigation of how the patient perceives the world about him, how he sees himself, how he uses what he sees and hears and smells, his memory, his thought processes, and all the emotional reactions that go along with thinking or with attempts to think. Next under our scrutiny comes the patient's behavior, what he does with his muscles. This must be examined both directly and indirectly. We must investigate what he does with his instincts, to whom he attaches himself and how he does it, what associations and connections and relationships he establishes, and what attitudes he develops toward himself as well as toward many parts of the outside world. All this takes time; it takes work. It requires examining, interviewing, psychological testing, and continued observation. It takes the collaboration of the members of a diagnostic team.

Obviously, psychiatric diagnosis is more than collecting data. It involves the organization of these data to provide answers to certain questions. The most important question, of course, is what form of treatment the patient should have. This was not always so. Diagnosis has come to imply treatment, but formerly it was largely a matter of giving a name to something recognized. Many people still think of diagnosis in this way, but this can be very misleading because, although knowing a name is *some* evidence of acquaintanceship, that acquaintanceship may be shallow or deep and there is no easy way of telling which. As acquaintanceship grows into deep understanding, names become less important; they may even be changed, and changed again. If the understanding is deep enough, names may be dropped altogether or replaced by adjectives such as "dear" or "darling."

Thousands of names have been given to the various forms of illnesses which people have observed in themselves and their friends or which physicians have observed in their patients. For a long time—we are not sure how long—people have suffered from conditions that we now call colds or fevers, measles or mumps, cancer or pneumonia. There are also many diseases that no one ever has any more, such as lycanthropy and typhilitis; there are some that few people now have, such as typhoid fever and leprosy. Sometimes this is interpreted as meaning that medical science has become the master of the situation. It is true that people no longer die by the millions of smallpox or the black plague. Today we have many miracle drugs which quickly abate the consequences of various infections. Preventive medicine and the whole concept of public health have made vast changes in the incidence of illness.

And yet sickness does not seem to disappear. Diseases keep disappearing, but sickness remains. It seems even to increase. Except in epidemics, doctors have never been so busy as they are now. Patients keep coming. Hospitals multiply, and they are all full of sick people. What does this mean? With what illnesses are these sufferers afflicted? What has taken the place of those potent enemies which have been slain by new discoveries or kept at bay by preventive medicine? What are people sick with today? What are the diagnoses?

The great paradox is that the patients who today crowd physicians' offices and fill hospital beds suffer, frequently, from conditions to which no simple diagnostic labels can be given. Their afflictions do not fall into the classical categories of illness. They do not correspond to anything in the textbooks. They do not fit the established entities. No standard names apply to them. These people are sick—there is no question about that. They are weak, they run fevers, they suffer pain, they lose sleep, they lose weight. All these and many other symptoms the doctors understand, for the most part, and handle with a high degree of proficiency and effectiveness. What the physician cannot do the surgeon often can. Infections, obstructions, inflammations, dislocations, paralyses, hemorrhages—all these we know, and we know what to do about them. But what are the diseases? What are the names for these illnesses?

The fact is that they do not have simple names because they are not simple things. The nature of illness has changed and hence also the meaning of diagnosis. A visit to a hospital will illustrate this.

For example, the man lying in room 417 is thirty-six years old. He has always been a frail chap, but he supports his widowed mother, with whom he lives. He works very hard in a large organization with which he has been associated since he left high school. Each day he immerses himself in the details of a tedious and complicated clerical job. From eyestrain, perhaps, or from sheer weariness, he developed intense headaches and, incidental to these, he lost time from work on several occasions. Upon the recommendation of an efficiency expert, payroll deductions were made for such sick leave; though not amounting to very much in cash, they gave rise to worry and sleeplessness in this man. He began to vomit after eating and hence to lose weight. Finally his frantic mother importuned him to go to the hospital, and here he is. The doctors have examined him. They found inanition, leucocytosis, and an enlarged spleen—nothing more. He seems to be improving. But from what disease? What is, or was, the diagnosis?

In another room in the hospital is a middle-aged, straight-laced schoolteacher, a little older than the first patient. She came to the doctor's office after school and waited her turn. She was frightened and tense. She described the intrusion of unpleasant thoughts from time to time which so occupied her mind as to impede her teaching activities. She lives alone, and has almost no friends or social contacts. Her principal had spoken to her about her depressed, worried appearance, and in fear of losing her job she had even considered suicide.

Hospitals and clinics alike are full of patients whose symptoms do not add up to the simple, clear-cut disease entities described in the books on the practice of medicine and there given official designations. "Clinical entities, while commonly appearing in case reports, do not exist in patients. . . . [They never help us] to understand the subtle qualities which lead to recovery in one and to death in another patient apparently suffering from the same 'entity.' " (2) Many conditions are given diagnostic labels which are almost nicknames. This man has a "back," this one a "heart," that one an "ulcer" or a "virus." These are not disease names, or even symptoms.

They do not precisely describe what the patient's trouble is. And what may we suppose these same conditions were called by the Trojans or the Hittites or the Egyptians, or even by our English ancestors a thousand years ago? Not to go back quite so far, what do you suppose they were called when I was in medical school, which was long enough ago? Something quite different, I can assure you.

Does this mean, you will ask, that each generation finds new names for old conditions? Or does it mean that the intrinsic nature of illness has changed? Are new diseases appearing to replace old ones, or do we merely understand the old ones better—or differently?

Perhaps all these things are true. Our understanding of illness has certainly changed, not once, but many times, since the days of Hippocrates. His model of illness as a thing in itself which entered or fell upon or developed in a victim was followed by physicians for hundreds of years. After they had wandered away from the original model, giving their attention rather to symptoms and their amelioration, Sydenham brought medical thinking back to the ontologic model. The discoveries of medical science in the next century helped to fill in some of the gaps in Sydenham's knowledge, and we made spectacular progress for a time. Fifty years ago we thought we knew the etiology, the pathology, the life history, and, in some instances, the proper treatment of hundreds of definite diseases.

Today we are not so sure about some of these things. We know effective treatments for many conditions, but we are less certain about etiologies. It would seem that most illnesses are more complicated than we used to think in the days when we could speak so definitely about various disease entities. Illness is to us today less an ugly visitor falling upon hapless victims by chance, than an altered state of being in an individual which has come about from the interaction of many factors.

Today in virtually every field of science the pattern of explanatory thinking is shifting from static, classificatory, single-cause analyses to dynamic, process-oriented, genetic explanations. Kurt Lewin has called it the change from "Aristotelian" to "Galilean modes of thought." [1] In such terms we can define illness as a certain state of existence which is uncomfortable to someone and for which medical science offers relief. The someone suffering may be the afflicted person or those around him or both, but a disturbance has arisen in the economics of an individual-environmental adjustment. The certain state of existence which is uncomfortable arises from this disturbance, this shift in balance. Shifts of some kind and degree are going on constantly, and with them constant processes of restoration. But certain events or combinations of events or persistence of events may upset the balance beyond immediate righting. Then comes a crisis, a state of emergency, and unusual restorative maneuvers are automatically instituted. It is the totality of these things, including the actual injury suffered and the form of the reaction to that injury or stress, which make up what we call the picture of illness.

This concept is based upon notions of internal and external equilibrium, the automatic maintenance of certain

---

[1] Lewin might better, perhaps, have called our modern modes of thinking "Heraclitean," bearing in mind the emphasis that Heraclitus and Empedocles put upon process, interaction, and conflicting forces.

levels of functioning within the organism by various homeostatic devices, first beautifully described by Claude Bernard
and later by Walter Cannon in biochemical and physiological
terms. These same concepts and principles can and, in our
opinion, must be extended to include psychological and social
factors. The interactions of individual and environment take
place in ways that cannot be adequately reduced to physical
and chemical terms. But organismic equilibrium maintenance
and reciprocation between the individual and the outside
world take place with the aid of special symbols, feelings,
gestures, thoughts, and acts, in patterns that are governed by
the same general principles of reciprocality and integration
which have been described by these eminent physiologists and
others in regard to body tissues and body fluids.

So, indeed, we believe. For us illness, as we use the
term in psychiatry, refers to precisely these broad considerations of homeostasis, of organismic equilibrium, internal and
external. When psychiatry was at long last gingerly incorporated within the peripheral confines of medical science, its
practitioners adhered faithfully to the orthodox dogma of the
parent body. They sought to discover disease entities corresponding to brain lesions of various kinds and loci. They applied names to their "discoveries." Even more than in general
medicine, an official label became the chief end of diagnosis.
It gave a sense of definiteness and partial security in an area
of great strangeness and mystery. It was a step forward when
Johannes Weir and his successors began to give names, however fictitious, to various forms of mental illness. It was a
move away from superstition. But disease names can come to
be regarded almost as were the witches before them, with a

kind of awe, unquestioning acceptance, and undying persistence.

As in witchcraft, psychiatric disease names came to be
pejorative and frightening. The very word "cancer" is said to
have killed, through fright, some patients who should not and
probably would not have succumbed to the malignancy from
which they suffered (1). The effect of some psychiatric words
can be terrifying and damning, even if not fatal. There is an
old aphorism about giving a dog a bad name and hanging
him. Obviously you cannot hang a good dog; he must first be
labeled "bad." We decide on the basis of his nature. One is
reminded of a passage in Lewis Carroll's immortal classic,
where the Knight has announced that the name of a song he
is going to sing is called "Haddock's Eyes." The following
famous conversation ensues:

> *"Oh, that's the name of the song, is it?" Alice
> said, trying to feel interested.*
>
> *"No, you don't understand," the Knight said,
> looking a little vexed. "That's what the name is called.
> The name really is 'The Aged Aged Man.' "*
>
> *"Then I ought to have said, 'That's what the
> song is called,' " Alice corrected herself.*
>
> *"No, you oughtn't: that's quite another thing!
> The song is called 'Ways and Means' but that's only
> what it's called, you know!"*
>
> *"Well, what is the song, then?" said Alice, who
> was by this time completely bewildered.*
>
> *"I was coming to that," the Knight said. "The
> song really is 'A-sitting on a Gate.' "*

One may look at the attitude of our ancestors toward mental illness, as well as the treatment methods it inspired, in several ways. Insofar as it was dictated by immediate self-interest and ferocity, it was a kind of defensive and hearth-guarding measure. To some extent it was an expression of the sadism or the destructiveness from which no one is entirely free, and which grows into dreadful evil when it can acquire some kind of social justification. One need only think of Cromwell, Torquemada, and the *apartheid* policy (not to come closer home).

But to some extent our ancestors must be given credit. They were trying to do something not only for themselves, but for the afflicted. Mercy was not entirely lacking. It was only that their concepts of illness—which we now believe to have been false—dictated a kind of treatment which was ineffective. Their study of the mentally ill in state hospitals, their attempts at the identification of various syndromes, their searches for causes with the logical consequence that many contributory factors were discovered, all helped to create a certain concept of mental illness in the nineteenth century which began to modify the philosophy of treatment.

Naturally, if there is a cause of something, that cause ought to be removed by logical means and not by the infliction of pain or the process of wearing someone out. And the cause of mental illness in the nineteenth century was pretty well agreed upon as defect in or damage to the central nervous system. Jacksonian twitches and jerks were known to indicate the presence not of witches but of brain tumors. The syndrome of syphilitic encephalitis became established as the classical and convincing paradigm of the brain lesion concept of mental aberrations.[2] Griesinger was the great exponent of the neurological concept of psychiatric illness, and in this sense was a "unitarian"; that is, he believed that various kinds of mental illness were only the reflections of various kinds of brain disease. This was not a new view; it was already prevalent in the eighteenth century when there was much less evidence for it. This evidence built up rapidly during the latter part of the nineteenth century, particularly through the development of brain-tissue staining combined with anatomical and neuropathological studies of many kinds. It will be recalled that Freud entered his professional career through the then popular field of neurophysiology, and almost discovered the local anesthetic effects of codeine. The clinical experiences of the Franco-Prussian and Civil wars added greatly to the clinical knowledge of brain localization. Clinical neurology was in its heyday. For the most part psychiatry was a kind of appendage made up of the epiphenomena of injury to the central nervous system.

Partly from the discoveries of Freud and Charcot; partly because of discoveries by Mesmer, Liébault, and Bernheim; partly from Ehrlich's discoveries of an effective drug; and partly from the experience in World War I with demor-

[2] Today we know, of course, that these syndromes may occur without spirochetal encephalitis, that most syphilitic infections of the brain do not produce the picture of "general paresis," and that the psychopathological symptoms of paresis sometimes respond to psychotherapy and not to spirochetecides. We know, in short, that syphilis alone does not "cause" the mental disorder "typical" of general paresis. Syphilitic and other toxins which injure the brain can contribute to the production of a variety of symptoms which in a given culture have a certain general similarity. But this is a far cry from our once cherished and "established" paradigm of a specific psychosis.

alized shell-shocked soldiers, dynamic psychiatry in the form we know it today began in the early part of the twentieth century.

Dynamic relates to the assumption that there are psychological pressures in certain directions and that these pressures stem from a complicated and interactive area of forces, partly intrinsic and partly extrinsic in origin. The dynamic concept of mental functioning, and hence also of mental illness, began to make serious inroads into the accepted thinking of psychiatrists about 1915. And although the "brain-spot-versus-mind-twist" issue continues to divide psychiatrists to this very day,[3] there has been a steady shift from the organic school, to which we all belonged some years ago, toward a dynamic position. Perhaps most psychiatrists would say that they recognize both concepts as applicable in varying degrees to every case. Unfortunately, however, textbooks, nosological designations, and legal statutes are all couched in the terms of the older concept, now considered by many obsolete. This explains how contradictory answers can be given in court by colleagues in good standing, who actually disagree, not regarding facts, but only regarding designations. This dispute goes further than merely professional disagreement. It has reached the point where conscientious and respected scientists openly refer to the "dishonesty" of equally conscientious and reputable colleagues. They refer not to financial skulduggery but to what seems to them a disloyalty to scientific principle—

---

[3] The issue is now complicated by a third, and even a fourth, position: the body-fluid concept of personality and disease, which is a kind of reversion to the old chemicalism of antiquity; and the Social Factor school, which is the ultrasociological and, in a sense, antimedical viewpoint.

in this instance, the principle that mental disease cannot exist without brain disease.

The proof of the pudding is in the eating, and the core of psychiatric diagnosis, that is, the concept of disease one holds, is the resulting attitude toward treatment. It is difficult to repair damaged brain tissue; hence, outside a few empirical methods of uncertain value, the organicists must rely on kindly care, chemical controls, and hope. How this attitude affected state hospital programs before 1950 need only be recalled— and recalled, indeed, without reproach. For, if one believes that treatment is useless and the outlook dreary, it is little less than charlatanry to go through idle and futile motions to impress the taxpayers and the relatives.

But here the dynamic school has a great advantage. For according to their theory—our theory—there is no foregone conclusion as to imperceptible brain damage. And, on the other hand, there are logical and rational indications for therapeutic intervention. This is the whole point of diagnosis. For those who can accept this newer viewpoint, psychiatric illness becomes hugely and splendidly treatable. The appropriate methods of inciting or assisting the self-corrective powers of the individual (and of the environment), and of throwing the weight of the physician's knowledge and concern on the side of the forces favoring recovery—this is what a proper diagnosis can show us. And this is the kind of diagnosis the patient wants, the relatives want, the judge wants. Not impressive name-calling, not pejorative classifications as sane or psychopathic or psychotic or eccentric, but a clear statement regarding the illness process: its general form, its present degree of severity, and its movement (trend). Appended to this is an analysis of the factors working for and against recovery, with an indication as to which of these is accessible to our efforts.

It is not a question of what names are used to designate an affliction, but of what can be done about it. What, and how, and by whom? This is the primary purpose of present-day diagnosis, to guide the form and the direction of the intervention. Treatment without diagnosis is charlatanry, but diagnosis without treatment is pedantry, and in the present state of world distress pedantry is even more reprehensible than charlatanry; it is the sin of indifferentism. For it is now accepted, not as an act of faith but as something clearly demonstrated, that there can be effective intervention in mental illness. There are ways to recovery. There is hope. For a long time no one believed it, and hence diagnosis had no such purpose. Today most psychiatric patients are cured. I said at the beginning that sickness is still rampant, that all hospitals are full and fuller. There is one great and pertinent exception: psychiatric hospitals are not fuller; they are slowly emptying. Their population is decreasing. In 1948 Kansas was about to spend $20,000,000 on a new institution because of overcrowding. For example, Topeka State Hospital, built for 1,500 patients, housed 1,850. No new institution was built and no new buildings were raised, and yet Topeka State Hospital today has 950 patients, many empty beds, and no waiting list.

Today no one doubts the efficacy of psychiatric treatment. Recovery is now expected, not merely hoped for. It is expected by the patient, the relatives, the physicians.

REFERENCES

1. CRILE, GEORGE, JR. A plea against blind fear of cancer (with comments by Drs. Evarts A. Graham, J. Englebert Dunphy, Charles W. May, Alton Achxner, and Walter C. Alvarez). Life, 38 (Oct. 31):128–142, 1955.
2. STEVENSON, IAN P. The constitutional approach to medicine. New York J. Med., 48:2156–2159, 1948.

3 HUMANISM AND

SCIENCE IN MEDICINE

BY GEORGE L. ENGEL, M.D.

IN RECENT YEARS it has become fashionable to stress the importance of the doctor-patient relationship and the necessity of considering the "patient as a whole," because of the fear that the humane aspects of medicine are being submerged by the emphasis on the scientific and the technical. Efforts are being made to modify medical curricula so as to enable the student to relate more to the patient than to the disease. In brief, physicians and medical teachers are again concerning themselves with the so-called "art of medicine."

These developments raise the question as to whether this interest in the doctor-patient relationship is a reflection of our humanism as physicians, or whether it has a specific scientific relevance for the course of disease and the maintenance of health. Do we want our patients to like and have confidence in us only because this is the way decent human beings should behave toward one another? Is it a matter of public relations and good press for the physicians, as some spokesmen of organized medicine claim? Or is it possible that between physician and patient there occur certain psychobiological processes (basic to human relations in general) which have significance for the capacity of the individual to maintain health or to develop disease? In brief, in respect to health and disease, is the bond between patient and physician a matter of science or of humanism? I propose that it is primarily a matter for science and, further, that the humanistic in medicine also has a scientific basis.

That the physician can exercise a healing effect without the exhibition of any specific treatment has been known and exploited by physicians throughout the ages. Indeed, so striking are the effects of physician on patient that one wonders how much this has contributed to the survival of medicine as a profession. What we know as scientific medicine is hardly a hundred years old, and even now specific curative remedies are few and far between. From time immemorial human beings have sought, found, and used healers, and it is this need of the suffering and the ill which has kept medicine as a profession alive through its millenniums of dark ages and into its present scientific infancy.

Is our understanding of health and disease sufficiently encompassing to take such factors into account? Disease is a condition of life; it is not something set apart. As Dubos has said, "The very process of living is a continual interplay between the individual and his environment, often taking the form of a struggle resulting in injury or disease" (8). Health and disease are relative concepts reflecting in essence the success or the failure of growth, development, and adjustment in a physical, biological, and social environment (25, 9, 10).

Psychiatry in Medicine

Departures from health or disturbances in adjustment are multidetermined. Simple cause-and-effect views of disease are no longer tenable. To quote Shimkin, "There are few, if any, simple or single causes in biology; there are instead complex situations in environments in which the probability of certain events is increased" (29). Our modern concept of disease must include all the parameters that bear on life itself, whether they are observable in physical, chemical, biological, genetic, morphologic, psychologic, interpersonal, or social terms. When considering how health is maintained or how disease evolves, we are no longer concerned with the single "cause," but with the necessary and sufficient underlying conditions. And the conditions of health and of disease are the conditions of life.

Once we have so broadened our horizons we discover a banality. Man lives by more than bread alone. Health and healthy development require certain kinds of experience and human contact over and above the other well-known essentials, such as oxygen, water, and nutriment. Indeed, terms like "nutriment" or "aliment" are sometimes used to identify the essential input to the mind, apparently necessary not only for its development but for the well-being of the whole individual (23, 24). This dependence on supplies from the environment is obvious enough to remain unnoted until a situation arises in which they are unavailable.

Then, as poets and philosophers have long informed us, profound changes in well-being may take place in the one so deprived, including even a decline to death. These matters have frequently been dealt with in spiritual, religious, or artistic terms, but scientists have given them scant heed. It is true that the great physicians, as sensitive observers of the human scene, were impressed with the significance of antecedents like despair and grief as possible factors in the genesis of many illnesses, including neoplasm, and stressed the role of faith and hope in recovery (20, 21). But with the explosive developments in scientific medicine in this century, interest in and awareness of such factors have been largely eclipsed by the contributions of the physical sciences. While tremendous new insights into psychology, stimulated by the discoveries of Freud, were evolving, the developments in biology and psychology, for the most part, remained unrelated. Now at long last it is becoming clear that a scientific basis exists for what has in past ages been known mainly through the insights of poets and of other intuitive, sensitive men. Now certain aspects, processes, and characteristics of the external environment are demonstrated to be assimilable by the developing organism, internalized, so to speak, and constituting conditions for living if not for life itself. The terms "objects" and "object relationships" are convenient for designating such phenomena. More specifically, objects (for humans) include not only other human beings, but also valued possessions, home, job, country, ideals, goals—that is, tangible persons or things in the environment as well as abstractions. Object relationship refers to the nature and the variety of interactions between a person and his environment which account for the objectivization of someone or some thing. Obviously, these processes are mediated by the central nervous system, and no doubt future study will reveal the nature of the underlying neurophysical and neurochemical events in the brain (18). But at the moment our most fruitful insights into these processes come through psychological studies and the observation of mental behavior.

How can we demonstrate the importance of objects and object relationships? The traditional technique in biology for exploring whether or not some element is necessary to life or to vital functions is to see what happens when it is not available or is in short supply. In respect to the essentialness of objects, this has long existed as an experiment of nature. I refer here to the phenomenon of grief, the familiar reaction to the loss of an object, whether it be a loved person, a valued possession, a job, a home, a country. Elsewhere, to emphasize the role of object relationships and the significance of loss of objects as conditions of life and living, I posed the question as to whether or not grief could be considered as a disease state in the same sense as pneumonia, a vitamin deficiency, a burn, or a neurosis (11).

Uncomplicated grief is a discrete syndrome which runs a consistent course modified mainly by the abruptness of the loss, the nature of the preparation, and the significance for the survivor of the lost object. When acute, it generally includes an initial phase of shock and disbelief in which the sufferer attempts to deny the loss and to insulate himself against the shock of reality. This is followed by a stage of developing awareness of the loss, marked by the painful affects of sadness, guilt, shame, helplessness, or hopelessness; by crying; by a sense of loss and emptiness; by anorexia, sleep disturbances, somatic symptoms of pain, loss of interest in customary activities, and impairment of work performance. Finally, there is a prolonged phase of restitution and recovery during which the task of mourning is carried out, the trauma of the loss is overcome, and a state of health and well-being is reëstablished.

Thus grief, like other conditions that we customarily think of as disease, involves suffering, an impairment of function and capacity to work, and an identifiable and consistent etiologic factor, namely, the real, threatened, or even fantasied loss of an object, and it has a relatively predictable symptomatology and course. The grieving person is often manifestly distressed and disabled to a degree quite evident to the observer.

Many find objectionable the inclusion of grief in the general category of disease. I have discussed these objections at length elsewhere (11). It is enough to say here that grief is the natural response to a loss in the same sense that a burn is the natural response to thermal radiation, or that typhoid fever is the natural response to the typhoid bacillus in a susceptible individual. That it is ubiquitous and in most instances self-limited, not requiring the ministrations of a physician for recovery, can be said as well of a host of other disease states.

Although the manifestations of grief are observable in psychological and behavioral terms, the absence of physiologic and biochemical changes during grief do not permit the claim that none occur. Actually, the matter has not yet been studied. That grief is not fatal is not only irrelevant but may even be untrue, at least if we are to believe the innumerable accounts, in literature and in the press, of individuals who have fallen ill and died in states of grief. Actually, the older medical literature is replete with alleged examples of this (20, 21), and we are beginning to find confirmation in current studies, as recently summarized by Schmale (28).

Even if the skeptic continues to find it difficult to link

the terms "grief" and "disease," no one can refute the reality of the phenomenon or the support it brings to the concept that objects and sustained ongoing object relationships, as defined above, constitute necessary conditions for the maintenance of the optimum condition of life which we refer to as health.

I selected grief because it is the most patent and glaring illustration of the consequence of object loss. It calls to our attention the necessity of learning more about the development of object relationships from early life onward, and about the role such processes play in the development of the mental apparatus and of the central nervous system. It raises questions as to how such processes may be connected with the psychological and social development of the individual, as well as with the regulation of the internal milieu. It calls for more precise identification of psychological and behavioral, as well as physical, expressions of changes in object-relating, for it is as important to know what occurs when objects are gained or object relationships are established as it is to know what happens when they are lost or disrupted.

There is a large psychoanalytic literature on object relationship, but in respect to the genesis of disease the work of my associates, William Greene, Franz Reichsman, and Arthur Schmale, has afforded important new insights. Schmale has pointed out that affects provide the most sensitive psychological indicators of the condition of object relationships and object-relating (28). Further, it is also clear that self-esteem, the intactness of the psychological perception of self, is enhanced in an important way by the nature and the status of the past, as well as by current object relationships and objects.

Schmale's work has indicated particularly the affects of helplessness and hopelessness consequent to object loss. Both these affects have their origins early in life, early in the development of the mental apparatus, and both bespeak the need for objects to maintain psychological integrity and intactness. Both are experienced subjectively as feelings of despair and discouragement which are concomitants of being let down, left out, overwhelmed, and so forth. Helplessness is perceived as coming from a change in relationship leading to a desire to be taken care of and protected by an object, whereas hopelessness is the feeling that no help is possible, that even if an object or a support from the outside should become available, it would not help because it is too late.

Whether or not one "gives up" consequent to object loss, be it real, threatened, or imagined, is determined by past as well as current factors, and cannot be predicted by the nature of the object lost or threatened. Grief therefore includes these affects only to the degree that the loss leads to "giving up," and the distinction between normal grief and unresolved grief in part reflects the capacity of the individual to deal with the loss and to substitute new objects for those lost.

The observations of our group, as well as of many others, suggest that when object loss is not successfully dealt with, more complex illnesses, including organic disorders, are likely to develop (28). And, as helplessness and hopelessness are the affect qualities indicating "giving up" consequent to object loss, so joy, confidence, hope, and self-esteem are the affects indicating successful, effective object relationships and the intactness of the self.

At this point it may be helpful to provide an objective

documentation of the nature of these states, and this can be done most conveniently through motion-picture studies of various responses of young children to object loss. Small children are better for illustrative purposes because more of the phenomenology is manifest in behavioral terms and therefore can be observed and recorded.

The first demonstration is of an eighteen-month-old boy who was entering the hospital for major surgery. This child was born with a congenital atresia of the esophagus, and in the first days of life a gastrostomy was performed, through which he has been fed ever since. The child has been under observation since birth, and the motion-picture record is available at intervals thereafter. He has been very attentively and devotedly cared for by his mother, who has rarely if ever let him out of her sight. In the film we first see a lively, active, curious little boy with his mother and father, busily exploring the room, running to and from his parents.

When both parents leave the room there is an immediate, frantic, tearful response. The child runs toward the door and reaches for the knob, crying loudly. This is unabated until the mother and father return a few minutes later, when the boy runs past the father to the mother, reaching out his arms to be picked up. Although looking somewhat somber, he is immediately comforted in the mother's arms.

The next scene demonstrates the child twenty-four hours later. He has been left in the hospital by the parents, whom he has not seen since. He is seated in the crib, his left hand holding a bar. He is almost completely immobile, his face is impassive, his lip corners are turned down, and he has a sad expression around the eyes.

The entry of a doctor whom he has known evokes little response beyond a slight turning of the head, with no vocalization. When the child is lifted out of the crib and placed on the ground, he is not only unsteady on his feet but walks with a shaky gait and with slow, mincing steps, and maintains his left arm and hand in the same fixed position, as if still holding the crib bar. He finally walks slowly to a chair and steadies himself with the left hand. When lifted up by the doctor he remains quiet and leans against him.

This striking behavioral change within twenty-four hours is interpreted as a depressive response to object loss, specifically to the loss of his parents, his siblings, his grand-parents, and his familiar home surroundings. The child seems overwhelmed, lost, in despair, helpless.

The third scene shows the child three weeks later, after recovery from a surgical repair and ready to be discharged from the hospital. His parents have visited him daily, staying for several hours at a time. The appearance now is of greater retardation and immobility than before. But when picked up by the doctor, who has also seen him several times daily, the child relaxes somewhat, though remaining relatively inactive.

When the mother enters the room he immediately reaches toward her with his arms and his whole body. Now, however, when held by the mother, he pulls away and cries vigorously. For the first several minutes she is unsuccessful in comforting him. This demonstrates the continuing impact of the repeated comings and goings of the mother and the significant change that has taken place, not only in his over-all behavior pattern, but in his mode of relating to the mother.

Additional information not recorded in the motion pictures revealed that for a number of weeks the child remained fretful, easily upset, and extremely intolerant of the mother's absence.

The second part of the movie shows a little girl, also born with congenital atresia of the esophagus and having a surgically produced gastrostomy. This case is described in detail elsewhere (12).

After this child was cared for by both mother and grandmother for the first six months, circumstances required the mother, with another small child, to separate from her own parents and live with her psychopath husband in a distant area. Depressed over this separation and again pregnant, the mother had serious difficulty in accepting and relating to her defective child. As a result there were long periods in which the little girl was neither held nor comforted, and in which she cried herself to exhaustion. In this setting, despite adequate caloric intake via the gastric tube, she failed to gain weight or to develop further, and even lost ground. At the age of fifteen months, when the first motion-picture recording was made, she weighed only ten pounds, was unable to sit up, and presented the appearance of marked marasmus and depression.

The movie illustrates this severe depression. After five months of attentive care, particularly by one nurse and one physician, the child showed a marked improvement, gaining weight, becoming responsive and attentive, and manifesting a full range of responsive behavior with pleasant, joyful recognition of both nurse and doctor. The old depressive behavior, however, was easily reproduced by the approach of a stranger when she was alone.

This was in contrast to the more usual and the expected anxiety pattern observed in children of this age and stage of development. The pattern included not only a profound immobility and hypertonus, the tendency to fall asleep, but also a marked reduction in gastric secretion, which became unresponsive even to histamine (13).

The movie also illustrates the child's immediate behavioral response and recovery on the return of the familiar doctor, and how, when a stranger accompanied the familiar doctor, the stranger quickly became associated with him and lost the capacity to provoke the depressive withdrawal response.

The second part of the movie provides evidence that a depressive type of response can develop in the presence of an object when the relationship is ineffective and, further, that this response can become a fixed pattern ready to be reëvoked under certain circumstances. The study also demonstrates certain significant biologic changes accompanying this state.

The movie is a graphic and convincing demonstration of the reality of the phenomenon under consideration. Spitz has amply documented the occurrence of such reactions among infants and has further described, under the term "hospitalism," the profound retardation in development when infants are brought up after the third month in a sterile environment with relatively few human contacts (30, 31). The "hospitalism" group suffered an unusually high mortality from infectious diseases. The whole field of the impact of early separations and deprivations among infants and small children is now the subject of wide interest (7).

What further is known of the consequences of object

loss when it is followed by "giving up" and by the affects of helplessness and hopelessness in adults? Here we are only at the beginning of exciting new insights. Over the past fifteen years there have been scattered allusions to the possible significance of loss, grief, depression, and so forth, as precipitating or conditioning circumstances for the development or exacerbation of certain specific diseases such as diabetes, tuberculosis, and thyrotoxicosis (28).

When unselected populations of medical patients were studied carefully from this point of view, this relationship was found to hold true in a number of conditions, as in leukemia, when no hint of such factors had previously appeared (16). Schmale finally studied a large number of unselected medical patients, the typical population found in the medical ward of a general hospital, and discovered a very high incidence of unresolved object loss, approaching 80 per cent, as an antecedent to the development or the exacerbation of the illness (28). Wolff, Hinkle, and their associates, using a different approach and a somewhat different terminology, were led to a similar conclusion: namely, that the state of giving up, with its corresponding affects, may be the psychological reflection of a more profound alteration in total biological function which serves to alter the capacity of the organism to resist or compensate for factors leading to disease (33).

Reports on the consequences of certain major social disasters seem to provide support for this view. Most notable, of course, was the appalling morbidity and mortality among American prisoners of war during the Korean War. With the destruction of morale and the marked dissolution of the pre-existing social supporting organization, the syndrome "give-up-itis" came to be recognized as an ominous prelude to serious illness and death. It was further noted that some soldiers could be saved if they could be stimulated into some kind of relationship, even an angry one, with a fellow soldier. In sharp contrast was the low morbidity and mortality among the Turkish volunteers, who for various reasons were able to maintain morale in highly effective interpersonal relationships (19). These reports are but more accurate and well-documented accounts of what has long been known among prisoners of war, concentration-camp victims, victims of disasters, or transported slaves. H. G. Wolff has recently summarized some of these observations (33).

Parallel with this are the fascinating autobiographical accounts of individuals who have survived such experiences. Strikingly apparent in all such accounts that I have read is the extraordinary capacity of the individual, not only to serve as an object for himself, but also to call upon his memory as an unending source of nutriment. Important, also, have been firmly held political or religious ideals or beliefs.

These observations only whet our appetites for more precise information. Naturally it is tempting to turn to the experimental laboratory where preliminary studies on animals are already rewarding. That animals exhibit grief reactions is well established and certainly well known by pet owners. Clearly here is a readily available source of experimental material for the investigation of biologic, biochemical, and physiological aspects of grief reactions.

The effects of early or previous experience on the susceptibility to disease is the subject of a growing literature. Time permits me to cite only a few examples.

It has been shown that the incidence of spontaneously developing mammary tumors in certain strains of mice is greater in animals living alone than in those living in cages with other animals (6, 22).

A recent series of studies has shown that the susceptibility to gastric ulcers in rats placed in a conflict situation is influenced by whether or not the animal is alone; an animal in the company of one or two others is more resistant (26, 27). Ader, using the same technique but experimenting on a strain of rats more susceptible to ulcer formation, failed to substantiate the protective effect in the paired situation, but he believes that the effect may have been masked by the greater susceptibility (3).

Ader was able to demonstrate, however, that the age at which infant rats were separated from their mothers had a significant effect on their susceptibility to ulcer formation in adulthood. Those separated at 15 days of age were significantly more susceptible than were those separated at 22 days (normal weaning time) and at 35 days. On the other hand, animals that had interrupted separations in the first 10 days of life (in contrast to the permanent separation at 15 days) were significantly more resistant than were the normally weaned animals (4). In other words, permanent early separation and interrupted early separations have opposite effects on the susceptibility of rats to ulcer formation when exposed to a conflict situation in adult life. That the increase in the susceptibility of infant rats separated at 15 days is not due to a nutritional deficit was demonstrated by showing that rats raised by a mother whose nipples were cauterized at 15 days were as resistant as the control (22-day) rats (1).

When susceptibility to alloxan diabetes was used as a dependent variable, preliminary data indicate that rats caged in groups of eight are more susceptible to the hyperglycemic effect of alloxan than animals caged individually (5). Paired animals, on the other hand, appeared to be more resistant than either animals alone or animals in groups of eight.

Another interesting finding has been reported by Groen (17). Hamsters are ordinarily gregarious animals and, when caged together, exhibit considerable body contact. If, however, a female hamster is successfully mated, and the mate is then removed and replaced by a strange male, the female will adopt a belligerent, threatening attitude, forcing the male to maintain his distance and a defensive posture. After some time, the male so isolated and threatened becomes manifestly ill and may die. In one case the autopsy revealed primary amyloid disease.

These studies strongly suggest that both early and current social relationships among animals are variables in the susceptibility to disease, and that this can be studied in the laboratory. The preliminary results from a number of different laboratories indicate that early-life experiences exert significant affects on the mode and the success of responses to later-life experiences, helping to determine what will constitute a stress and the capacity of the animal to deal with it. Biologic factors, on the other hand, determine the nature of organic defects that evolve under such circumstances. Thus, in rats subjected to physical restraint, significant variables underlying the susceptibility to erosions in the stomach include strain, sex, and the level of plasma pepsinogen (2). Surely here is an enormous field for future research, not only further to elucidate the role of such factors in disease, but also to discover the biochemical and physiological processes involved.

Whether we concern ourselves with man or with animals, what engages our attention is the significance of the internalized (learned) aspects of the environment which serve regulatory functions for the organism. What we have designated as object loss is essentially some change in the "fit" between this internalized environment and the real external environment. Most often this is brought about by a change in the environment, as caused by a death or a separation. It may also come about, as psychoanalytic studies have amply demonstrated, from internal, psychologic changes, so that the environment seems different, as in a fantasied loss.

In either situation, however, it is well to emphasize that we are identifying a ubiquitous psychological stress. This means that the concept of objects and of object loss is meaningful mainly in terms of the existence and the operation of a mental apparatus. Whatever the consequences of object loss, whether manifest ultimately in biochemical, physiological, or social terms, the change in the environment must first have been perceived and apperceived and the consequences mediated by the central nervous system. This imposes upon us the necessity of paying more attention to the role of the central nervous system in the maintenance of the functional integrity of the organism as a whole, as well as of its parts. This neglected field is now beginning to attract much interest. Stewart Wolf, in his Minot Lecture of 1959, reviews some of our current knowledge in this area (32).

Finally, we come back to the implications of these developments for the care of the patient. We are proposing that the mysterious ingredient, the powerful therapeutic influence of the physician, the hospital, the clinic, the placebo (not to mention nonmedical or paramedical healing influence), is none other than the effect of a substitute object. When, to the high frequency with which illness is preceded, if not precipitated, by object loss (real, threatened, or fantasied) and depression, we add that any illness or disability may provoke object loss secondarily, the potential importance of object replacement becomes obvious.

Some years ago I suggested that the doctor may be seen as fulfilling "a surrogate ego role" for the patient (14). This is perhaps simply another way of formulating the processes discussed in this paper, as we now recognize the role of object relations in developing ego function and can understand better how object loss may bring about ego regression. Whether the physician operates as as "surrogate ego," or whether he serves as an object and thereby brings about more effective ego function, is less important than our recognition that the doctor-patient relationship may be a key factor in achieving the mental and emotional stabilization of the patient.

It is of interest that the word "confidence" describes the affective state most representative of the optimal conditions for survival and growth both of the child in relation to his mother and of the patient in relation to his physician. Obviously, confidence alone is not enough, for, as we well know, confidence may be misplaced, in physician as well as in mother. This, however, is not the place to elaborate on the subtleties of the factors underlying the relationship of physician and patient, which psychoanalysis has elaborated in terms of transference and countertransference. Rather, we wish to emphasize the significance of the physician's successfully fulfilling the role of object for the patient.

From all this the conclusion seems inescapable. The humane care of the patient, in all its aspects—how the doctor, the nurse, or the attendant behaves, how the hospital is run, how the operating room or radiology department functions— must have a rational scientific basis. That which is humane is humane because it takes into account the scientific bases underlying human relationships, especially in the object- relating aspects. When the humane is based on maudlin sentimentality, on "do-goodism," on the principles of public relations or advertising, on sympathy rather than empathy (15), then it may as often deviate from as coincide with a sound scientific basis. In that event it may have disastrous consequences.

The major thesis of this paper is far from proven. It is, to some of us at least, highly suggestive and certainly exciting. I have tried to provoke more critical consideration and to stimulate new approaches to investigation. I want to emphasize the pertinence of John Romano's warning that the present problem of medicine is not that it has become too scientific, as some claim, but that is has not yet become scientific enough (25).

REFERENCES

1. ADER, R. Unpublished data.
2. ADER, R., C. C. BEELS, and R. TATUM. Blood pepsinogen and

gastric erosions in the rat. Psychosom. Med., 22 (no. 1):1–13, 1960.

3. ADER, R., C. C. BEELS, and R. TATUM. Social factors affecting emotionality and resistance to disease in animals. I. Age of separation from the mother and susceptibility to gastric ulcers in the rat. J. Comp. Physiol. Psychol., 5 (no. 3):496, 1960.

4. ADER, R., C. C. BEELS, and R. TATUM. Social factors affecting emotionality and resistance to disease in animals. II. Susceptibility to gastric ulceration as a function of interruptions in social interactions and the time at which they occur. J. Comp. Physiol. Psychol., 5 (no. 3):455, 1960.

5. ADER, R., and H. L. JACOBS. Social factors affecting emotionality and resistance to disease in animals. III. Reactions to alloxan in group and individually caged rats. To be published.

6. ANDERVONT, H. B. Influence of environment on mammary cancer in mice. J. Nat. Cancer Inst., 4:579–581, 1944.

7. BOWLBY, J. The nature of the child's tie to his mother. Intern. J. Psycho-Anal., 39 (no. 5):1–24, 1958.

8. DUBOS, R. Mirage of health. New York, Harper, 1959.

9. ENGEL, G. L. Homeostasis, behavioral adjustment and the concept of health and diseases, *in* Mid-Century Psychiatry, ed. R. Grinker. Springfield, Ill., Charles C. Thomas, 1953. Pp. 33–59.

10. ENGEL, G. L. A unified concept of health and diseases. Perspectives in Biology and Medicine, 3 (no. 4):459–485, 1960.

11. ENGEL, G. L. Is grief a disease? A challenge for medical research. Psychosom. Med., in press.

12. ENGEL, G. L., and F. REICHSMAN. Spontaneous and experimentally induced depressions in an infant with a gastric fistula. J. Am. Psychoanal. Assoc., 4 (no. 3):428–451, 1956.

13. ENGEL, G. L., F. REICHSMAN, and H. L. SEGAL. A study of

an infant with gastric fistula. Psychosom. Med., 18 (no. 5): 374–398, 1956.

14. ENGEL, G. L. The surrogate ego role of the physician in the management of physically sick patients. Round-table discussion of psychotherapy in medical and surgical hospitals, midwinter meeting, Am. Psychoanal. Assoc., New York, Dec. 8, 1951.

15. ENGEL, G. L. Affects in terms of drive, ego, and self-object, a developmental perspective. To be published.

16. GREENE, W. A., JR., and G. MILLER. Psychological factors and reticuloendothalial diseases. IV. Observations on a group of children and adolescents with leukemia: an interpretation of disease development in terms of the mother-child unit. Psychosom. Med., 20:2, 1958.

17. GROEN, J. J. Personal communication.

18. JOHN, E. R. Some speculations on the psychophysiology of mind, *in* Toward a definition of mind, ed. J. Scher. Glencoe, Ill., Free Press, 1960.

19. KINKEAD, E. In every war but one. New York, W. W. Norton, 1959.

20. KOWAL, S. J. Emotions as a cause of cancer. Psychoanal. Review, 42 (no. 3):217–227, 1955.

21. KOWAL, S. J. Emotions and angina pectoris. Am. J. of Cardiology, 5 (no. 3):421–427, 1960.

22. MUHLBOCK, O. F. E. Invlaed van bet millieu af de kunkerontwikkeling. Onderzalkingen by de melkklierkanker van de muis. Ned. Tydschr. v Geneesk, 94:3747–3752, 1950.

23. PIAGET, J. The construction of reality in the child (1937). New York, Basic Books, 1954.

24. RAPAPORT, D. The theory of ego autonomy: a generalization. Bull. Menninger Clinic, 22:13, 1958.

25. Romano, J. Basic orientation and education of the medical student. J. Am. Med. Assoc., 143:409, 1950.
26. Sawrey, W. L., J. J. Conger, and E. S. Turrell. An experimental investigation of the role of psychological factors in the production of gastric ulcers in rats. J. Comp. Physiol. Psychol., 49:457–461, 1956.
27. Sawrey, W. L., and J. D. Weiss. An experimental method of producing gastric ulcers. J. Comp. Physiol. Psychol., 49: 269–270, 1956.
28. Schmale, A. H., Jr. Relationship of separation and depression to disease. Psychosom. Med., 20 (no. 4):259–275, 1958.
29. Shimkin, M. B. *In* Cancer, ed. R. W. Raven. London, Butterworth and Co., 1952, p. 162.
30. Spitz, R. A. Hospitalism, *in* The psychoanalytic study of the child. New York, International Universities Press, 1945. Vol. I, pp. 53–74.
31. Spitz, R. A. Anaclitic depression, *in* The psychoanalytic study of the child. New York, International Universities Press, 1946. Vol. II, pp. 313–342.
32. Wolf, S. Natural integration and the mechanisms of disease. Minot Lecture to the Section on Internal Medicine, Am. Med. Assoc., Atlantic City, June 9, 1959.
33. Wolff, H. G. The mind-body relationship, *in* An outline of man's knowledge of the modern world, ed. L. Bryson. Garden City, N.Y., Doubleday, 1960.

4 THE HUMAN APPROACH

BY DOUGLAS D. BOND, M.D.

THE WORD "human" is ordinarily a synonym for kindly, understanding, or compassionate. The word may be used, however, in its opposite sense: for example, to explain the faults, the cruelties, and the frailties of our race we may say, "After all, he's only human." The complex antithetical meanings of the word reflect the complex antithetical nature of man himself.

Is there any other approach of a physician to his patient than a human and, in this sense, a compassionate one? In a common wish to return to "the good old days," there is a popular belief that the old-fashioned physician knew the family well, delivered the children, set the bones, listened with patience, counseled wisely, and never sent a bill. He might well have done so, for there was little else for him to do. The number of patients he saw was relatively small, his armamentarium was simple, his overhead was low, and his clientele had a wholly different idea from today's of what the physician could or should do. For one thing, the patient was likely to feel fortunate that any doctor at all was available.

Good health was not claimed as a right; it was considered a privilege.

Patients were not apt to visit the doctor as a result of feeling a little tired or of having an irritating wife or husband. With travel restricted, the chance of seeing more than one doctor, and therefore of obtaining conflicting opinions about treatment, was slight. The patient had no choice, and he was careful not to demand too much for fear the physician would fail to come when he next needed him. Public knowledge about disease was scanty, and the doctor's word reigned.

All this has changed. Patients can and do drive many miles to the physicians of their choice. Medical knowledge has advanced, and specialists abound. Studies and treatment of patients are complex and expensive, and involve many people other than physicians. A relatively sophisticated clientele of today knows a great deal—not only about common diseases like cancer, heart disease, arteriosclerosis, and neuroses, but even about multiple sclerosis, amyotrophic lateral sclerosis, and the various muscular dystrophies—and demands more. Patients frequently know a good examination from a poor one, a shotgun treatment from a specific one, and an excessive use of diagnostic studies from a critical use. Whereas, on the one hand, knowledge builds strength and lessens useless fear, on the other it lessens blind faith and sharpens criticism. The doctor is required to know more, to treat more, to see more patients, and his added burden tends to dehumanize him.

With the increased importance of knowledge there has been a decreased emphasis on charm, on patience, and on comprehensive understanding of the patient. The idea old-fashioned physician never had to try to learn all there was to know about the patient and his family; he simply could not avoid learning it.

Have we swung too far toward faith in the laboratory, the X ray, and the EKG? The claim that we have seems to result from two factors: (1) the scientific conclusion that the lives and the minds of people play an intimate role in bodily health; and (2) the public image of the physician, no longer the kindly old philanthropist but a busy younger doctor who refuses to make house calls, insists on Wednesday afternoons and Sundays off, drives two large automobiles, sees that his bills are sent out on time, and has a collection agency to police his accounts. A peculiar part of the myth of the doctor of bygone times is that he was always old, never young and bustling. The public image does not let today's younger men grow older, any more than it lets the proverbial family doctor start young.

In 1912, when Flexner made his study of medical schools in this country, there were approximately 175, most of them proprietary. They were run for the profit of the teachers who saw that the less they spent on pupils and the more pupils they had, the more profit they made. Laboratories were practically nonexistent in most of these schools, and cadavers were few. The two-year schools, which prided themselves on being superior to the one-year schools, often merely repeated the same course in the second year. It is hardly likely that these schools—and the bad ones far outnumbered the good—turned out many men who by any stretch of the imagination could be compared with the physicians of today. A physician of those times was likely to bleed or purge patients, and often carried infection from one patient to another. The body's own balancing force was a far better healer. Kindliness and gentleness, good sense, keen observation, and conservatism in the use of the therapeutic tools then at hand were a physician's best equipment.

Only very recently—indeed, within the twentieth century—has the physician become truly effective. It is true, of course, that even in the old days there were exceptions; some physicians were ahead of their times. The rise of physiology and then of biochemistry has given us an enormous impetus toward understanding how the body works and toward finding clues to help the sick. Though knowledge now is incomplete compared to what it will be, it is monumental compared to what it used to be.

With the new breakthrough, the attention of physicians has swung sharply ahead. The hope of having tools that will make for real effectiveness is a heady one, but all the tools are not yet at hand. The hopes are partially premature, for man is a complex animal. Pneumonia can be cured, but there is still much to be learned about treatment for alcoholism, for irritable and straying husbands, for bed-wetting, and for back pain that worsens after removal of the uterus. The back pain may be the one escape left from a feeble-minded child or an alcoholic husband. When alcoholism graduated from a defect in character to an illness, the doctor's burden became heavier.

To rise to the challenge, the doctor must keep his special status. If he is to have a practice rather than a business, he must meet the new demands with perspective, balance, and compassion. He must not let himself lose the gentle touch. He must make himself listen; he must fight cynicism; he must empathize with his patient. He must control his own anxiety and his own frustration. He needs to feel effective, to feel that he can help solve any problem brought to him. Because of the hopes of universal effectiveness, a certain kind of physician feels defeated when a patient does not respond to treatment. But patients do not apply to him in order that he may prove his skill. His job is clearly to heal when he can, but otherwise to comfort. It is unfortunate that in some large medical centers a hopeless patient is told, "There is nothing more we can do for you."

Not long ago, the mother and the brother of a young woman dying of multiple sclerosis came to see me in my capacity as dean of the school. They inquired whether the patient's donation of her brain and spinal cord to the medical school would really advance the knowledge of this disease. Unless it did they preferred to withhold the gift, because it interfered with the accustomed burial rites. We settled the question and, as the brother stood up to leave, he told me that the neurologist had sent this patient home with the statement that there was nothing he could do for her. The patient, who liked and respected the doctor, became severely depressed. Telephone requests for the neurologist to visit her were of no avail. Finally the brother burst into his office and demanded that he visit the patient regardless of expense. The doctor came, and the house was transformed. The patient became cheerful. The whole family situation became tolerable. The doctor thereafter visited the patient for fifteen minutes once a month. The brother, who had forced the doctor to make the calls, said to me: "Is this really the way medicine is taught and practiced? I don't think it's right."

A fine man in our community developed a malignant melanoma of the nose which metastasized to his spine. He wrote a widely reprinted article entitled, "I Have Cancer." In response to this courageous statement he received thousands of letters from all over the world. He surprised his physician, who came to see him regularly, by asking, "What are my chances?" The doctor was embarrassed but replied, "Only a miracle can save you." Then followed a period of severe hysteria in which the patient's wife joined. The patient was upset; he could not sleep or enjoy a moment's comfort. His friends encouraged him to report to them on the land between life and death. Finally, somebody suggested that cancer was a psychosomatic disease and that, as I was a psychiatrist, I ought to be called to treat him.

It was at this most unfavorable time that I entered the scene. I told the wife that her husband's seances with his curious friends must stop, that it was clear he was going to die soon, and that I might help him to settle down, though I could do nothing more. From that time until he died, three or four months later, I visited him two evenings a week, and he told me about his life. My constant response was that his life had certainly been interesting, and that I would see him in another few days. When his time came, the man died like a man and not like a baby, and I felt that my evenings had been well spent.

In psychiatry we seem to develop the idea that we should push every patient out of the hospital regardless of how ill he is, as if this were in itself an achievement. It may be extremely easy to discharge patients from hospitals, but this is no criterion of a hospital's excellence.

Some years ago, in another city, I was asked to discuss the case of a seventy-year-old army nurse who had been in the service thirty or forty years. Both her husband and her only child had died. She had no relatives and almost no friends.

One evening she was quite depressed while walking along a street. A handsome and courteous gentleman doffed his hat and asked if he might accompany her home. She immediately saw him as someone to be trusted, and she began to take painting lessons from him. It seemed to her that he was a savior come to her rescue, and she knew he had given her the most precious gift in the world. She continued to paint, but after a while she became violently upset, fearing that her neighbors were trying to steal her paintings because of their great value. She turned her hose on her neighbors, and, on the day of her admission to the hospital, called a locksmith ten times to change the locks on her doors.

The young man who presented this case said he had tried dissembling therapy, which had failed, and he now wondered if the patient should not have a lobotomy so that she could be discharged from the hospital. Dissembling therapy, I learned, meant that a patient could have delusions and hallucinations but could be taught to keep them to himself. It was no surprise that this treatment had failed. What would be the point of being selected for this great recognition and then not being allowed to tell anyone, especially when one was lonely and abandoned? The purpose of the whole psychosis was to avoid the depression of loneliness. If this psychosis were taken away from the woman, with what could it be replaced? The light on her face when she told her story made it apparent that it gave her enormous pleasure.

A mental hospital is a place where people understand such a patient, and do not scoff at her private solution to her dilemma; where she can be cared for; and where she will annoy a minimum of other people. To provide such an environment for such a person ought to give a great deal of satisfaction. I would feel far from kind if I were to assault her and her psychosis in order to improve my statistics.

My approach to built-in homeostatic mechanisms in the mind and body should not be considered as antitherapeutic or antiscientific. When the physician takes into account the reasons for symptoms, in many instances he will forego a therapeutic attempt and will give comfort as he can.

5 ECOLOGY AND

THE SPIRIT OF MAN

BY STEWART G. WOLF, JR., M.D.

IN THE JUNGLE PERIOD man's way of life was predominantly competitive. His major health needs were food and protection from wild beasts and the elements. At some time in this period man made the great discovery that he could achieve his ends more quickly and more effectively through coöperation than by relying solely on his competitive nature. Thus societies were born. The effective creation of a society required that males, accustomed to mutually destructive sexual conquest, would have to learn to live together peaceably. It has been suggested that this circumstance brought the loin cloth into existence, as a device to play down sexuality so that men could work together. To enable men to work together, social groups were formed. As groups, however, they continued the pattern of competition and the efforts at mutual extinction. A part of the world was overrun now by one group, now by another. The major hazards to health during this period were pestilence, poverty, and malnutrition.

More recently there has been added a further refinement of civilization: the functions of the individual have become highly specialized so that the interdependence of people has become obligatory. The needs of the human infant had shown that it was imperative to care for others, but one may assume that some little time passed before such a relationship was recognized as applicable to adults.

Within the new social groups, larger than the former tribes and nations, there came about the need for almost total curbing of promiscuous hostile and sexual drives. Thereupon diseases of a psychological and psychosomatic character came into prominence. Before man had any real conception of society, the appropriate way to deal with an opponent was to kill and eat him. The linking of gastric hypersecretion of acid and pepsin with circumstances arousing hostility and resentment may have been an appropriate adaptation gradually established (perhaps through mutation) over thousands of years.

During the past few thousand years, however, as man's conception of society has changed from a primary emphasis on competition to a greater concern with the benefits of coöperative living, his altered behavior has left no enemy flesh in his stomach and nothing for his digestive juices to work on but his civilized meals and his own tissues. While the old, slow evolution of natural selection still obtained, the great discovery of the utility to coöperate in effect added a new evolutionary dimension. Man found that his way of life could evolve more rapidly through the exercise of his powers to decide and to communicate with his own and subsequent generations. He was no longer dependent on mutations.

The design of man's body, still dependent presumably on the slow mutative process, has not kept pace with the demands of human ingenuity. Our respiratory and circulatory apparatus are not geared for flight into space. In fact, our adventurous spirit has faced us with an environmental challenge comparable to the one that was met by the first aquatic animals that ventured onto dry land. It is already clear, however, that it will not take man so long to adapt to the ether as it took fishes to move safely into the air.

There is some evidence that a change is occurring in man's digestive apparatus. Pepsin seems to be the universal protein-digesting enzyme in the gastric juice of all meat-eating animal forms, from fishes on up. Man, however, has in his gastric juice, in addition to pepsin a second protein-digesting enzyme which operates effectively in a less acid medium than does pepsin. Why should there have been the need for so much acid in the stomach? Of course, animals had the habit of eating bones, and highly acid juice was needed to decalcify the bones. Man has not eaten bones for many thousands of years. His second enzyme, capable of digesting the meat in a less acid juice, may represent a mutative adaptive process. At the moment we seem to be in midstream from the standpoint of evolution, because man still secretes both enzymes, pepsin and gastricsin. We have been searching among medical students for one whose gastric juice contains only gastricsin. He would represent, of course, an advanced species of human development, an evolutionary blue blood. It would then be interesting to study the gastric juices of members of his family. Whether or not man can learn to adapt to his fellows in a healthier way before the destructive pepsin and the hyperacidity of peptic ulcer are eliminated through mutation we do not know, but it will be interesting to watch.

What has psychiatry provided to solve this and other similar problems of medical ecology? I believe that efforts to understand human nature have placed a disproportionate emphasis upon the more or less negative characteristics of man. Very properly, but perhaps one-sidedly, psychiatry has been facing problems arising from the need to suppress and sublimate primitive drives, and the difficulty of self-expression with guilt arising from normal needs and pressures. There is good evidence from the paintings in the caves of Cro-Magnon man, twenty-five to fifty thousand years ago, that man's most primitive needs include something on the gentler side.

There has been comparatively little concern with man's aspirations, his aesthetic needs, his thirst for knowledge, and his love of virtue.

When altruism has been recognized in animal forms, including man, many psychologists and psychiatrists have passed off the manifestations somewhat lamely as sick exaggerations of restraints or vicarious gratifications of a basic instinct. The facts of history do not really bear out this negative interpretation. As C. P. Snow said in *The Two Cultures and the Scientific Revolution:* "It is a mistake which anyone who is called realistic is especially liable to fall into, to think that when we have said something about the egotism, the weaknesses, the vanities, and the power-seekings of men, we have said everything. But they are sometimes capable of more. And any realism which doesn't admit of that isn't serious."

It may be that the positive nourishment of the spirit of man may contain an important key to his health and growth. It may be, indeed, that we will find that altruism is a hard, practical asset, just as coöperation turned out to be. Altruism may provide a third dimension to evolution and accelerate even further man's quest for his goals. It was certainly a great discovery when animals first learned that they could protect themselves by exterminating one another. When it was learned that coöperation had more survival value than competition, a really startling contribution to progress had been made. It may be that generosity of spirit has even more power. There is certainly widespread evidence that a primary concern for the welfare of others leads to greater comfort and satisfaction for the party of the first part. Isn't this what happens when an organization has superb morale? Or in the many human situations where superior teamwork wins?

Man's brain is capable of integrating an enormous amount of information from his surroundings and his experiences. It deserves more and more study by those interested in human behavior. Behavioral science is still a fledgling. We need more, not less, science. We must understand the emotional needs of people, individually and collectively, and we must learn more of the significance of deprivation.

Our behavior is largely patterned by the decisions we make, consciously or unconsciously. Our capacity to elect among various alternatives a certain course of action implies that we have a system of values. Many of man's values are based on needs of the spirit far removed from the need for personal survival, food, and sexual gratification. Many of his emotional conflicts and pangs of conscience probably derive from his failure to adhere to his scheme of values and to gratify his gentler needs. According to Ogden Nash, "There is only one way to happiness on this terrestrial ball—that is to have a clear conscience or no conscience at all."

There is ample evidence that the nourishment of the spirit is relevant to bodily health and performance. At Western Electric, when the company officials wanted to find out whether fluorescent lighting would increase the efficiency of working girls, they installed it in one of the workrooms. The productivity of the group working in that room soon exceeded the productivity of all other groups. Then it was suggested that the girls might do even better if the walls were painted a pastel shade. That worked, too. Really interested by now, the management decided to test the effect of increasing the height of the workbenches by six inches. Again productivity increased, but then it was discovered that lowering the workbenches by six inches had the same effect. Ultimately it became clear to the officials that what was helping these workers toward better achievement was the recognition that someone was interested in their welfare and comfort.

Another famous experiment was carried out by Frederick the Great in a foundling hospital in Germany. To cut down the mortality rate by eliminating germs, insofar as possible, he ordered the hospital attendants to change the babies' linen frequently, to keep things scrupulously clean, and to feed the children promptly but without holding or cuddling them in any way. Thus he hoped to avoid communicable diseases. Surprisingly, however, the lack of human warmth and loving resulted in the death of most of the babies, although at autopsy there were no specific lesions discernible.

How often have we seen the broken spirit of an aged person lead to his deterioration and death when he no longer felt wanted or useful. Dr. Calvin Plimpton, the president of Amherst College, tells the story of a man who died and shortly thereafter found himself transported to a delightfully cool and comfortable spot where his every want was supplied as soon as he mentioned it. In fact, one of the angels, who appeared to be assigned to him, continually asked him what he would like to have in order to raise his level of enjoyment. He asked for, and received, a fine house with a kidney-shaped swimming pool, a fine car, and a few fine young ladies, as well as a few rather prosaic luxuries. He was having difficulty in deciding just what else he desired, when one day he asked, "Isn't there some work I could do around here?" The angel replied, "Oh, gracious, no! There's no work." "Well, couldn't I be useful in some way? Isn't there something I could help out with?" There seemed to be no opportunities along this line at all. Becoming more and more restless, the man kept imploring the angel for some little thing he might undertake in the way of work, but always with the same reply. Finally in exasperation he said, "Well, if it's going to go on like this indefinitely, I would have preferred to go to Hell." "And just where," said the angel, "do you think you are?"

The study of the lofty aspects of man's spirit ought to prove as interesting and as fruitful as the study of his more earthy qualities. In fact, this might be the new frontier for psychiatry.

6 PSYCHODYNAMICS

BY FELIX DEUTSCH, M.D.

PSYCHODYNAMICS is a field in which I have roamed scientifically for more than forty years. You will, therefore, rightfully anticipate that I approach it as a clinician and as a psychoanalyst. A few examples chosen from the past and the present may illustrate how I became, and still remain, interested in the research of psychodynamic (or psychosomatic) processes.

My interest was first aroused through experiments on guinea pigs. The sciatic nerve on one hind leg of a guinea pig was cut and, after a latency period of several weeks or months, whenever the cheek on the same side was pricked or squeezed the animal reacted with convulsions. Observation revealed that the cheek on the operated side was covered with lice, which the animal could not remove by scratching because the sciatic nerve had been cut on that side. The helplessness against the itching, which created emotional irritability, induced an epileptic seizure. When the skin was cleaned of lice, the squeezing of the cheek produced, not a convulsion, but only a light reflex spasm, or no reaction at all.

In animals exposed for a longer time to the epileptoid condition, however, only a slight touching of the trigeminal area sufficed to provoke a seizure. Why? Was a memory imprint established, a psychodynamic process that could not be extinguished? It resembled a conditioned reflex.

Analytic investigation (1921) of the conversion symptom provides evidence to support the theory that, when a traumatic effect is repressed and becomes unconscious, the repression leads to a symptom formation which lasts until the repression is lifted. To demonstrate this I conducted a hypnotic experiment on a female patient whom I knew to have a particularly strong attachment to her mother.

While she was under hypnosis, I suggested the following to her: She has gone for a walk with her mother in the surrounding woods. The sky is clouded over, but she does not notice that and continues walking ahead of her mother. Looking behind at a crossing, she fails to see her mother and runs back, but loses her way. She thinks she can hear her mother call anxiously. There is thunder and lightning, and darkness comes on. She stumbles and falls, tries to get up, and finds that she has hurt her foot and can walk only with difficulty. Suddenly, in the darkness, she thinks she sees a shadow beside her. She tries to escape from the shadow, loses her purse and her handkerchief, and runs back to look for her handkerchief. She hears a rustling in the bushes and starts off in another direction, losing her way still further. She becomes panicky. Finally she sees a clearing in the woods and runs toward it. The thunderstorm lets up. She reaches the clearing and is overjoyed to see her mother on the other side. Mother and daughter are reunited.

Throughout the time I was making these suggestions, increase in pulse rate and elevation of blood pressure were recorded. She was then given the posthypnotic suggestion that she would feel all right after awaking; that, whenever I took my handkerchief out of my pocket, she would experience the same anxiety she had felt in the hypnosis when she lost sight of her mother; that this feeling would disappear when I put my handkerchief back into my pocket; and that in neither reaction would she know what she was afraid of. She was told, however, that the whole memory of having lost her mother would be recalled when I dropped my handkerchief to the floor.

Upon awaking from hypnosis, the patient reacted with marked palpitations, anxiety, and feelings of oppression every time I drew my handkerchief out of my pocket. These feelings were noticeably stronger than those she had shown during hypnosis, and indeed they steadily intensified.

I then dropped the handkerchief. This produced a memory of an outing with several friends, whose names the patient was able to recall. There were no other recollections but, as she reported these fragmentary thoughts, her agitation decreased. I again dropped my handkerchief. The patient then recalled, as if it had been a reality, that a thunderstorm had occurred once during an outing with her mother, that she had lost a handkerchief, and, finally, that she had become separated from her mother but later had found her again. These memories came slowly and hesitatingly, and were expressed with agitation. After the recollections the exposure of the handkerchief produced no further anxiety. The anxiety and the vasomotor disturbances vanished when the repressed memories of a traumatic emotional experience become conscious.

Another observation demonstrates that if too much time has elapsed after the occurrence of such an experience and its repression, organic and emotional imprints which conscious recognition cannot remove may remain.

Forty years ago a patient came to me, complaining of difficulty in walking because of severe pain in his right foot. The pain had begun quite suddenly a year earlier, and he felt as if his foot were no longer alive. His physician had diagnosed a claudicatio intermittens, and had even considered amputating the foot. Because it was possible to establish collateral circulation, the thought of amputation was abandoned. Whatever therapeutic measures were undertaken resulted, however, in only temporary improvement. The circulation in the artery involved never returned to normal. When all attempts to treat the condition had failed, the patient began to wonder if it might be due to nerves. His illness, he recalled, had begun on the day of a major emotional upheaval. His pains had begun a short while after he left the hospital where his young nephew had died. The objective signs in the leg of this thirty-five-year-old man were in accord with the history. The pulse of the right dorsalis pedis was not palpable; the right foot was colder to the touch than the left. There were no demonstrable changes elsewhere in the vascular system.

When all medical measures proved of no avail, I decided to analyze the patient. The analysis eliminated his symptoms as soon as the structure of the psychodynamic process was made conscious. The question was: What kind of psychodynamic process had led to this symptom information? What was the content that had to be repressed, and, finally, when did this process begin to develop?

The analysis revealed that one reason for the patient's walking difficulty was his impotence. He had never mentioned it to his previous physician. His unconscious argument was, "As long as I am not potent I can't walk." At times he would have to stop in the middle of the street to tie his shoelace tighter, because of his feeling that the affected foot hung limp inside his shoe. His foot appeared to symbolize the penis. Moreover, on the day his nephew died—a death that he, who had no children, had wished for—he had hoped to have proof, through an extramarital venture, of his potency. Because of his nephew's death, however, he could not keep the rendezvous. "Better not to walk at all, than not to walk there," said the voice within him. Hence his inability to walk was a punishment for his death wishes. From then on the patient suffered from a limp, made still more obvious by his compulsion to touch small pieces of paper and other objects on the street with the bad foot, as if to examine their "mysterious" content. This habit added to the clumsiness of his gait.

The disturbance in his gait had still another cause. Almost fifteen years earlier he had read somewhere that "intermittent claudication is a very puzzling, mysterious disease." The sentence had remained in his memory, and he kept trying to feel the pulse in his foot artery. The sense of mystery, however, was not related to this illness alone. His unconscious incestuous wishes for his mother, which became conscious in his analysis, had to be repressed. Female genitalia always meant to him something "mysterious," with full knowledge forbidden. This was expressed for a long time in his ignorance of this part of the female anatomy. His limp was also partly due to his identification with his mother, who herself had a slight limp. As a result he himself had always been conscious of his own gait, particularly as a child. Finally it was revealed that the choice of the foot that limped was based on yet another childhood event. One time, when his mother was passing through the room, he tripped her with the same foot involved in the present illness, and she fell. The recollection was accompanied by a strong sense of guilt; his need for punishment, at any rate, was striking.

These antecedents provide, to be sure, a well-founded explanation of the psychodynamic process. It may be assumed that in the development of any psychogenic disturbance the part of the body involved must show a compliance that is both psychic and organic. This is a viewpoint repeatedly mentioned by Freud. The fact that organic changes may be brought about by psychic events is thus particularly emphasized. As the lowering of the water level in one of two communicating tubes leads to its rise in the other, so the relationship between psychic and organic factors is determined. The more the symptom is supported by one, the more easily can it dispense with the support of the other.

The organic determinants in this case soon become apparent. The patient had a limp because of the closure of an artery. Does this represent simply a leap from the body to the mind? Did the vascular disturbance of the foot become fused with the psychic apparatus without intermediary events? We must guard against such assumptions, just as we must guard against the danger, as Freud always warned, of bringing actual psychic traumata into too close a connection with conversion symptoms.

The patient showed a considerable eosinophilia. Was it due to psychic or to organic causes? I was already inclined at that time to think that the eosinophilia was of psychogenic origin, and, in the course of the analysis, without any other medical intervention, the changes in the blood cells disappeared even before the muscular spasm itself ceased. Our present-day knowledge of the effect of psychic stress on the adrenal cortex provides some explanation for the manifestation of eosinophilia in the course of some emotional disorders.

During the analytic procedure we depend almost exclusively upon the verbalization of thoughts and feelings. Very often we become aware of preverbal behavior, apparently related to the psychological situation of the moment. Sometimes the patient spontaneously expresses bodily sensations which he perceives and which can be interpreted as belonging to a psychosomatic unit. By and large, however, we tend to forget that analysis, which stirs up large quantities of psychic energies, is continually accompanied by correlated invisible physiological adaptations and responses. It should be kept in mind that whatever happens in one part of the organism is reflected in the whole and motivates the function of the whole. This is true for the simplest as well as for the more complex processes. Some reactions may escape direct observation and inconspicuously become established as specific patterns of behavior. By and large, their habitual response to external influences remains unrecognized. According to the "law of the psychosomatic unit," invisible bodily behavior is integrated into the psychosomatic pattern just as visible behavior is. These behavior patterns, formed as the result of experiences in the biological and psychological development of the individual, may become fixed. Certain psychosomatic skin disorders seem to result from such mechanisms.

Simultaneous photoelectric and mechanical plethysmographic recordings from the finger tips of both hands show that a physical as well as an emotional stimulus applied to either side of the surface of the body evokes a reaction on both sides of the body. The photoelectric-plethysmographic tracing may be used for the study of a number of phenomena. As the absorption of light by transilluminated tissue varies with its blood content, vascular changes of the skin may be detected. One may observe the rate and the rhythm of the pulse as well as changes in pulse volume. Ordinarily an increase in pulse volume accompanies an increase in finger volume, and a decrease in pulse volume is accompanied by a decrease in finger volume. Every change in the blood volume in one finger pad is simultaneously reproduced in the corresponding finger of the other side and becomes manifest as mimetic synchronous waves. Some patients always show a steady curve of blood volume. Others have very unsteady curves, with many fluctuations which are believed to be the result of unconscious emotional stimuli.

A cold stimulus applied to the back of one hand, until the sensation of cold is perceived, provokes a mimetic response on the other side. The degree of mimetic reaction is independent of the reaction on the stimulated side. Very often the vasoconstriction expressed in the decrease of finger volume and pulse volume precedes the actual perception of the cold sensation. This suggests that the vasoconstriction is not, or at least not fully, a reaction to cold as such, but rather an unspecific response to a stimulus, because the speed of the reaction is too rapid for the intervention of hormonal or chemical factors. It is likely that the response to cold has a neurogenic reflex basis similar to the psychogenic waves and is ideationally provoked. These mirrorlike vasomotor reactions seem to be unspecific, for they are not provoked by the particular stimulus itself on the rest of the body. The responses in other parts of the body may therefore be ideationally motivated. Some evidence of this assumption may come from the following observation.

F. G. was a forty-year-old, white, married man, whose first symptoms of lichen planus appeared twenty-three years ago, when he attended the funeral of his mother. She had suffered for years from tuberculosis. He suddenly felt itching on his left arm, with which he had lifted his sick mother out of and into her bed. On those occasions he had very often, to his embarrassment, felt her naked body. He used the hand of the same arm for sexual practices on his own genitals, and on this arm he had experienced twitching and beating movements as a child. He had once broken the arm. It is significant that his mother, to whom he was deeply devoted and with whom he identified himself in many respects, was left-handed. Her death was a hard blow for him. He had ardently prayed that her life be saved, although she had asked him to pray for her death. He developed a phobia about driving a car, as he was afraid of hitting somebody, of having a collision, of killing himself, or of meeting with some other catastrophe. He also believed there was a poison in his body and that he had to keep himself thoroughly clean. This led to a compulsive washing ritual. The skin condition of his left arm was of particular concern to him.

The plethysmogram of the patient at rest showed a rather steady curve with few respiratory waves. A cold stimulus applied to either hand led to a decrease in finger volume. This reaction was considerably stronger on the left side; even when only the right hand was stimulated, the reaction on the left was stronger and more protracted than on the stimulated side. When sense perception of cold and pain had disappeared subjectively and objectively, a spontaneous aftereffect occurred which resembled the reaction to the original cold stimulus. Later associations of the patient to the sensation on the hand suggested that it was the reaction to a kind of afterimage, expressing defense against a repressed unconscious wish related to the touching of the mother's genitals. This aftereffect of the cold-pain stimulus was further expressed in waves of decrease in finger and pulse volume, which were symmetrical but dissociated, as the decrease in finger volume on one side was accompanied by an increase on the other side, and vice versa. Furthermore, the disquietude of the curve on the left side lasted longer than that on the right side. It appears that tissue predisposed to irritation takes a longer time to subside after responding to a stimulus. This unusual reaction varied in intensity on different days when the experiment was repeated.

The simultaneous plethysmographic study on both finger tips of this patient revealed that the cathexis of a part of the body may lead to a dissociated vasomotor behavior. This was brought to the fore by the application of different stimuli to the skin.

THEORETICAL CONSIDERATIONS

The role of unconscious motivation in human behavior can be predicted. It is based on the assumption that a person's total make-up and probable reactions at any given moment are the product of past interactions between his specific genetic endowment and the environment in which he has lived from conception onward.

Freud applied the term "psychodynamics" to a process whereby a disturbing idea is rendered innocuous by transmuting the excitation attached to it into some bodily form of expression. He demonstrated that this mechanism was in the service of "the constancy principle." For example, repression of an erotic idea is accomplished by attaching the affect to some part of the body and thereby developing a symptom.

In his *Three Essays on the Theory of Sexuality,* Freud distinguishes between sexual (id) and nonsexual (ego) energy: "We distinguish libido in respect of its special origin from the energy which must be supposed to underlie mental processess in general." He used the term "sublimation" to describe the process of development in which the energy of infantile wishful impulses is not cut off but remains ready for use. Psychic forces are set in motion by external or internal pressure which interferes with the discharge of drives and thereby brings about an inner conflict. The internal pressure associated with the conflict or with the frictions between masculine and feminine strivings can mobilize dynamic forces. The term "drive" includes and presupposes a dynamic process.

The ego needs dynamic forces for its function. The drives in question are the erotic and the destructive drives. If the sexual drives go too far with their demands, they will be desexualized under the influence of the destructive instincts, whereas a too-high degree of aggressiveness will be lowered (disaggressivized) by the increase of libidinal drives. The psychic energies used in these processes have their physiologic counterparts.

The dynamics of personality consists of the way in which psychic energy is distributed and used by the id, the ego, and the superego. Once the energy furnished by the instincts has been channeled into the ego and the superego by the mechanism of identification, a complicated interplay of driving and restraining forces is activated. All prolonged tension stems from the counteraction of a driving force by a restraining force. Whether it be an anticathexis of the ego opposed to a cathexis of the id, or an anticathexis of the superego opposed to a cathexis of the ego, the result in terms of tension is the same.

If the work of the mind consists of a psychological activity such as thinking, it is perfectly legitimate, Freud believed, to call the form of energy used, "psychic energy." According to the doctrine of the conservation of energy, energy may be transformed from one state into another, but is never lost from the total cosmic system. It follows that psychic energy of the body and of the personality (or mind) is the id plus its instincts. An instinct is defined as an inborn psychological representation of a biological drive. The psychological representation expresses itself as a wish, and the bodily excitation from which it stems is called a need. An instinct is a quantum of psychic energy or, as Freud put it, "a measure of the demand made upon the mind for work." All the instincts taken together constitute the sum total of psychic energy available to the personality. An instinct has four characteristic features: a source, an aim, an object, and an impetus. The aim is the removal of the bodily excitation.

When the energy of an instinct is more or less permanently invested in a substitute object, that is, in one that is not the original and innately determined object, the own body, the resulting behavior, is said to be an instinct derivative. The displacement of energy from one object to another is one of the most important features of personality dynamics. Freud's theory of motivation was based solidly on the assumption that the instincts are the sole energy sources for man's behavior. Although Freud did not pretend to know how many instincts there are, he classified them under two general headings: life instincts and death instincts.

Personality develops in response to four major sources of tension: (1) physiological growth processes, (2) frustrations, (3) conflicts, and (4) threats. Symbolization, identification, and displacement are three methods by which the individual learns to resolve his frustrations, conflicts, and anxieties. They are also methods by which he may regain an object that has been lost. If psychic energy were not displaceable and distributive, there would be no development of personality. A person would be merely a mechanical robot driven to perform fixed patterns of behavior by his instincts.

Under the pressure of excessive anxiety, the ego is sometimes forced to take extreme measures to relieve the pressure. These measures are called defense mechanisms. The principle defenses are repression, projection, reaction formation, fixation, and regression. All defense mechanisms have two characteristics in common: (1) they deny, falsify, or distort reality; (2) they operate unconsciously so that the person is not aware of what is taking place.

The ego is said to obey the reality principle and to operate by means of the secondary process. The aim of the reality principle is to prevent the discharge of tension until an object that is appropriate for the satisfaction of the need has been discovered. The reality principle suspends the pleasure principle temporarily because the pleasure principle is eventually served when the needed object is found and the tension thereby reduced. The secondary process is realistic thinking.

Psychoanalysts firmly believe that a well-balanced psychodynamic process depends on the harmony of the id, ego, and superego forces. This concept does not undervalue the importance of complementary characteristics of environmental objects or of events which may exert their influence (provided they are well timed and favorable for their retrojection) in accordance with the ego-id-superego balance. The ego must have sufficient time to withstand the great demands of the id as well as the threat of the superego forces at all levels of development. In my opinion, however, the chief emphasis lies in the way in which sensory functional processes necessary for the awareness of reality are projected onto and inextricably tied to objects, and how after the cathexis of these objects they are retrojected onto the body, where they remain symbolized and dormant, thereby influencing the vacillations of the physiological processes.

My implications from Freud's conceptualization of

visual dream images involves a chain of events which begins with a physiological sensory perception leading to symbolization, in turn stimulating the physiological processes, which in turn revive need-gratifying objects in a hallucinatory way. When need arises, an impulse or a wish seems to recathect the object. The first memory is established only by gratification, which stops the impulse. I have pointed out that fundamentally psychodynamic processes may occur in any organ according to its erogenicity, and that they are composites of functional bodily disorders on different levels. The ego alters the function of an organ when its erogenicity and its sexual significance increase. The pathways leading to the symptom formation are well defined, and the psychophysiologic process is active long before the actual symptom is established. The psychodynamic process as the formative agent is based on the necessity to ward off emotional tensions; it results in a transformation of libido into the soma. The total somatic function is a reflection of a continual psychodynamic process which attempts to adjust the individual's instinctual drives to the demands of the culture in which he lives.

There are eight different stages of this process:

1. It begins with a loss by the child of an object (mother body environment) as soon as it is born.

2. The first awareness of this loss creates a fantasy or illusion as an attempt to regain the lost sensory perception by imagining it.

3. All external objects are perceived by the child as if severed from his own body.

4. The insatiable wish for the reunion with the

lost body, once initiated by a purely organic event (birth), is continually revived by a psychodynamic process of a different kind, where imagined and real losses of an organ or a part of the body became the representation of the lost object. It is this reunion that I named "retrojection."

5. The physiologic functions of the body parts that have become the representatives of these objects are modified because of a fundamental psychodynamic process.

6. The purpose of the psychodynamic process is to retrieve through retrojection the lost body and to maintain the body unity.

7. The wish to redeem the object by retrojection often overcompensates for aggressive feelings, and may lead to alteration of physiologic function; these feelings are the most important roots of the death instinct, which is an essential part of the ambivalence conflict. The wish for destruction contained therein is directed from the objects one wishes dead unto one's own self.

8. When one form of the psychodynamic process fails to achieve its goal, that is, to prevent anxiety, the ego must use other defenses to maintain integrity.

Therefore, the psychodynamic process is itself complex. The beginning is at the earliest period of life, when the ego is rudimentary and does not use sexualized energy. It is identical with the primary process. It originates in the need to replace an imagined and symbolized loss of body integrity. Organ symbolism is unconscious in a waking state, just as knowledge of dream symbolism is unconscious in a dreamer's mind. Some authors do not accept this concept because they feel that a psychodynamic process which takes the form of a conversion may occur before the development of a certain degree of ego structure. Others place more emphasis on the conscious part of mental activity and claim that the conversion process may be used either by the primary or the secondary process.

Margolin emphasizes that, insofar as one's conception of the operation of the body and its parts is derived by sensations and subjective experience, one may speak of "phantasy of function." In general, these fantasies of function undergo continuous modification under the abrasive influence of reality testing. Fantasy of function is different at various stages of development. It is especially marked at the psychophysiological transition points such as weaning, bowel training, speech and motility training, puberty, and adult sexuality. Thus, Margolin states that a succession of fantasies of function becomes a part of the unconscious. But he agrees that the psychic representation of an organ can and does undergo enormous modifications according to the genetic development and the experiences of the individual. He feels that in this respect psychosomatic disorders are the result of what he calls "a psychophysiological regression." Archaic fantasies of function return as psychophysiological components of mood and bring about infantile autonomy of organ functions. Because of low body tolerance, decompensation and disability result. Hendrick likewise feels that unconscious fantasies of patients give us invaluable information as the specific nature of the crucial conflict, but do not show why the tensions lead to a dysfunction in a specific organ. His hypothesis is that the choice of organ system is the result of "physiologic infantilism." His principle of physiologic infantilism in the somatization process is explained by the tendency to discharge conflict in those organs where the physiologic lability of normal immaturity has been retained or can be established.

Most of my co-workers in our former workshop group, like Avery Weisman, feel that the form of the psychodynamic process depends as much on the kind of fantasy which is repressed as upon the processes of conversion, symbolization, and retrojection. Hence the repression of certain parts of the fantasy content is of crucial importance, and when this is symbolized certain unmotivated visceral and somatic functions which participate in the performance of the act may be altered. The crucial question of the psychodynamic process, as with all defense mechanisms, is whether or not the particular process or mechanism can be correlated with any specific stage of ego development or libidinal development.

It seems that in the course of the psychodynamic process the more immature ego defenses are body-oriented. Mann and Semrad feel that, particularly in the psychotic, the psychodynamic process affects the ego development earlier than in the neurotic.

The specific nature and content of repressed fantasies at all levels of libidinal development play a vital role in the quality of the psychodynamic process. The ego may alter the function of an organ when either its erogenicity or its aggressive significance increases. The symbolized object is then always retrojected in a partially damaged state in order that symbiotic needs motivating the processes may be perpetuated. Exacerbations in the intensity of psychodynamic processes, as well as symptom development, occur when the attempt by the ego to release bound energy attached to the retroject clashes with the demands of superego forces.

It seems appropriate now to raise the question whether we are today nearer to the doorstep of the once-utopian hope of putting the edifice of analytic metapsychology on a biological foundation. Recent anatomical and physiological studies have implied that it is the diffuse reticular core of the central nervous system which exerts a vital, tonic, regulatory influence on the sensory systems, thereby modulating incoming sensory data in accordance with the central state of the organism or the behavioral significance of the stimulus.

There already exists anatomical and electrophysiological evidence that there are direct neural pathways from the highest central level of sensory projection, the cerebral cortex, back to sensory relay stations of the somasthenic system. The electrical activity of individual second-order nerve cells may be directly excited or blocked by neural activity generated in the same sensory cortical area to which these cells project. Spatial (somatotopic) relations are preserved throughout the system. Such a system might operate so as to (1) refine the attributes of sensation, (2) organize perception, (3) form the early stage of mnemonic processes, (4) set the receptive tone of the modality, or (5) initiate phenomena in the absence of peripheral stimuli.

This raises hopes that a structure has been found which makes it possible, with some justification, to put the psychoanalytic edifice of the personality make-up on a biological foundation. Such a structure may fulfill the once-utopian hope of closing the gap between the mind and the body. The reticular formation may constitute "the primitive mass," the mass of small cells interposed between sensory and motor components. This formation has been shown to have important relationships to sleep and wakefulness. It is a network which taps the sensory system and feeds into the motor outputs of other structures, thereby intervening in the automaticity of the functional systems. It can, so to speak, focus attention on a particular channel of sensory input of motor activity for the purpose of making new pathways.

It appears that more anatomical substrata of consciousness are located here than in any other place in the brain, because unconsciousness is most frequently associated with damage here. This ability to prevent the intrusion into consciousness of information, characteristic of alertness, appears to be a function of the reticular system, not only through action at neighboring relay stations but also through newly elucidated feedback systems which suppress the information not relevant at the given time. Penfield has suggested that corticifugal impulses from all sensory areas in the cortex are integrated by the reticular activating system into memory patterns, and projected back again to the cortices of the temporal lobes, where they are stored more or less permanently. This throws a completely new light on the psychodynamic processes and facilitates a comprehensive approach to the problem of psychodynamics.

In conclusion, physiologic studies, though incomplete, suggest that the brain-stem reticular formation influences both sensory input and motor output. Evidence has related these reticular pathways to autonomic control, neuromuscular function and, especially, to subserving the attributes of "consciousness." This latter function underscores the role of the RAS in clinical psychiatry. As stated concisely by French: "The reticular activating system must be considered the great integrating mechanism of the brain without which unity of response to complex environmental stimuli is impossible." Stated simply, this system contains the basis of the conscious awareness that permits man to react appropriately to his environment.

One of the exciting implications to be drawn from current laboratory studies is that the reticular formation is possibly one of the anatomic substrates for perception, and perception is the fundamental process that must underlie all the activities that characterize mind.

7 THE EMOTIONAL

PROBLEMS OF AGING

BY MAURICE E. LINDEN, M.D.

IT HAS BEEN suggested in this symposium that we need more science in current civilization. I believe I understand this concept. But I admit that I find myself growing more sentimental as I grow older, and my personal experience seems to be corroborating a hypothesis I put forward nearly a decade ago: as an individual matures, the normal aspects of his ego grow less egocentric, less narcissistic, and more altruistic (2).

Four years ago, in the same mood, I wrote the following (1):

> There is probably no better preparation for training in the field of gerontology or geriatric psychiatry than a visit to a Home for the Aged. Expecting to witness the classical stigmata of old age, the student will watch for the syndrome of social superfluousness, generally regarded as characteristic of the advanced years: mental deterioration, confusion, disorientation, loss of contact, memory impairment, and deficient per-

sonal hygiene. He will look for the signs of senility and of psychophysical degeneration. Thus armed with the platitudes and preconceptions of society, the student will find, instead, that he has entered a world apart— a special world, different from his expectations.

Coming from a world of motion, novelty, intrigue, ambitiousness and conflict, he will discover himself transplanted into one of meditation, reflection, discourse, philosophy and pathos. Instead of the cackling hag of legend, he will encounter the doting mother telling proudly and fondly of the activities and successes of her brood. Instead of the hollow-eyed, gaunt and wizened specter of a superannuated man, he will find a robust and busy little chapel sexton who stopped counting the years after he passed 80. He will meet a prettily dressed and lovely female septuagenarian waiting on tables and saying that she would darn and knit too, if only her eyesight were better. He will see an exhibit of expressive paintings by a man who will boast of never having had a paintbrush in his hand until after he retired. As he walks through the halls and wings of the Home, the student will hear a learned discussion of an obscure philosophical passage in the Bible; a peroration delivered with passion and braggadocio on the all but lost crafts of the flea market; a vivid description of the ancient art of waiting and buttling; a comprehensive consideration of the factors that lead mankind to war; a perceptive inquiry into the components of good family life. He may well witness the committee working in preparation for next Friday's party, hear a debate on the engineering achievements in the new crop of automobiles, or the implication of automation in the future of man. He is in a world apart; a world of reverie, critical consideration, thought and deliberation. This is the world of the older mind.

The foregoing description of aged persons is at variance with generally held social attitudes toward this group of people and highlights the bias and prejudice which lie at the foundation of popular opinion. The tendency to refer to them as "seniles" connotes hostility. Only a portion of the people of advanced maturity are truly senile. Indeed, a very large number of the aged have emotional problems related to aging, but in the strict sense not precisely caused by it.

Owing to the recent White House Conference on Aging (January, 1961) and the widespread focus on health care of older people, the problem of aging and of the aged has acquired a tone of respectability. Now every state in the Union and all the service agencies are developing programs and systems of care for the country's 16.5 million people over sixty-five years of age.

The increase in interest in older citizens does not yet reflect a similar increase in knowledge of or concern about their psychological problems. There is still a marked tendency to regard the problems of oldsters merely as the problems of youngsters grown older. Stemming from this notion is the logical belief that any therapist or practitioner who possesses skill in the management of the emotional problems of any other age group must, perforce, be competent to deal with older people. This idea, though slightly true, is mainly in error.

If any member of the healing arts desires to be an effective therapist with older people, he must view them as much more than simply familiar organisms grown older and in decline. He must, indeed, see the oldster as (1) an outgrowth of his culture, the recipient of prevalent attitudes, and hence a member of a sociologic group; (2) the logical culmination of a massive aggregate of lifelong intrapsychic phenomena, and hence an individual with specific neurotic needs which arise out of childhood, are influenced by fortuitous experiences, and are augmented by reactions to the special stresses of aging; and (3) the product of cumulative biologic alterations and psychophysiologic events, and hence a person with physiological needs and limitations.

WISDOM OF AGING

At this juncture let us consider, in accordance with psychologic concepts, the social value of wisdom, which is regarded as the essential gain of aging. A philosophical excursion into the meaning of wisdom may in fact parallel our psychologic notions very closely. Bertrand Russell, when recently asked to define wisdom, said: "It is a word concerned partly with knowledge and partly with feeling. It should denote a certain intimate union of knowledge with apprehension of human destiny and the purposes of life. It requires a certain breadth of vision, which is hardly possible without considerable knowledge. But it demands, also, a breadth of feeling, a certain kind of universality of sympathy." This definition, though incomplete, is a superb working hypothesis in which we may find bases for new concept formations.

Dr. Russell's first concept word is "union." As he uses it—"union of knowledge with apprehension of human destiny and the purposes of life"—it may be translated into psychiatric terminology as almost identical with "integration." Integration means the union of related forces through interdigitation, approximation, association, merger, combination, interweaving, and attachment. Both union and integration denote a smooth relationship among coöperative forces.

Russell's second concept word is "knowledge." In psychiatric terms, "knowledge" is identical with "fund of information." It constitutes the yield of several dynamisms: (1) formal learning through rote memory; (2) learning through experiencing, including the concepts of "emotional impact" and "resolution of conflict"; (3) information gained through a logical process in which parts of a whole are perceived and the remainder (the Gestalt closure) is conceived; (4) invention, in which ununited ideas are interacted to yield a novel notion not hitherto experienced.

The third concept phrase Russell uses is "apprehension of human destiny." Apprehension is prediction, the foretelling of events. The process of prediction is intimately related to past experience. The resolution of a prior problem becomes the content of a forecast when identical or similar problematical circumstances are presented. Just as "those who do not remember history are doomed to relive it," so, it may be surmised, those who do remember history may apprehend coming events. In this sense apprehension of human destiny is a logical process which represents the combination in thought of rote memory, recollection of conflict, emotion attached to the conflict, experience of resolution, and the rational yield of a likely pattern of future human circumstances.

The fourth concept phrase, "the purposes of life," covers value judgments, opinions, attitudes, philosophical considerations, and invented and learned ideals, aims, and goals, which together are equivalent to "meaning," an essentially rational process.

The fifth concept, "a certain breadth of vision," must in psychiatric terminology relate to two specialized concepts: (1) the depth and scope of inner and outer perception through awareness at various levels of consciousness; and (2) the availability and the mobility of psychological energies such as interest, curiosity, inquiry, and attention. Such energies may coincide with the concept of nonsexual libido. Dr. Russell's belief that breadth of vision requires "considerable knowledge" suggests that the panorama of perception is enlarged in direct proportion to the extent of resolution of prior conflict.

The sixth and last concept is "a breadth of feeling, a certain kind of universality of sympathy." Here I believe Dr. Russell has introduced the realization that human wisdom, which relates so intimately to an understanding of the vicissitudes and tribulations that face all mankind, implies empathy, mutual identification, and introjection. In other words, Dr. Russell is saying that the perceptive ego is simultaneously (1) aware of prior experience, (2) aware of conflict at some level,

(3) capable of solving conflict, (4) capable of lateralizing and externalizing the new experience to embrace other acting egos, and (5) capable of arriving at resultant solutions involving a mass of egos through an empathic matrix that predicts further interactions.

My purpose in performing this exercise with Dr. Russell's concepts is to demonstrate that the development of wisdom is the function of the growing, unfettered ego. Our common sense would tell us that aging is a small problem to egos capable of integrating knowledge and human feeling into a breadth of vision which apprehends human destiny and the purposes of life. And that is precisely what our experience and our researches are teaching us. All of us know many people —colleagues, friends, acquaintances, or patients—for whom aging will not be especially difficult. Of them we say, "They are too vital, too vigorous, too alive to be overconcerned with mere aging." Aging to them is another challenge, another circumstance to be negotiated, a new experience. They prosper as they continue to love life and living.

In an analogous manner, we are acquainted with people who, we believe, are so healthy and strong psychologically that they will never suffer nervous breakdowns. They possess enormous ego strength and great inner resources which enable them to resolve conflicts and survive social deprivations. They possess a richness of inner feeling and thought so that, even in situations of personal isolation, they are far from lonely.

To people like these, the worst of growing old is the possibility of a chronic physical ailment, such as arteriosclerosis, or of simple senility. They will, however, continue to function adequately, without being a nuisance to others, until such time as they become physically incapacitated.

In my experience, individuals who suffer great difficulty in the process of aging have always been emotionally frail. For them the psychological problems of growing old constitute "the last straw," which triggers the onset of a psychosis or a neurosis hitherto merely postponed. In such instances mental illness has already existed for many years, but has been overlooked, or tolerated, until intensification in later years causes the oldster's behavior to become unpleasant to those around him. Usually "problem oldsters" have been problem youngsters who fortuitously escaped serious disorders until the exigencies of aging could no longer be denied. Yet the skills required for the treatment of younger people do not necessarily carry over to the treatment of oldsters. A new set of understandings must be added.

The vaunted wisdom of the aged, in accordance with our reasoning, is the growing personality wealth and adaptability found in well-functioning, integrated egos. Individuals thus gifted make their own way in the world. They emerge as leaders and social examples, as well as preceptors to the young. Such people do not need public or welfare services, but, on the contrary, are more apt to give them.

But for the bulk of humanity, the great horde of people who emerge from childhood development still smarting from the humiliation, the suppression, the belittlement, and the wounds to pride they suffered in infancy, aging is fraught with serious obstacles. Their psychological resources are still too intimately bound to the business of keeping inner defenses intact. Their mental energies are not free to roam the broad exciting vistas of interpersonal living. They view life with gun-barrel vision. New factors introduced into the areas of their blind spots become massive impediments for which they are ill prepared.

My continuing studies of the aged are leading me to the conclusion that there is an increasing normality among people as they grow older. We often ask, "What happens to untreated neuroses in the period of aging?" The answer may be that they have become intensified, and show up as huge obstacles to aging. In the main, however, these neuroses consist of collateral channels into which unacceptable and intense instinctual energies have driven the reluctant ego. Clearly a neurosis under such circumstances is a subterfuge for dealing with overwhelming instinct which tends to be alien to the ego's orientation. In the course of aging, it is often noted that one of two events appears to be taking place in the individual who is not so beset by his instincts: either the instinctual drives have diminished and make less insistent demands upon the ego, and thus mitigate the need for a neurosis; or, if the instinct continues essentially unabated, the experiences of a lifetime may lead the primitive energies into sublimations. Whatever the intrapsychic mechanisms, many people actually become mentally healthier as they grow older.

SOCIAL REJECTION

The biologic decrements and physiologic alterations that become intimately associated with disease processes representing the logical culmination of chronicity tend to produce a need for intensification of old defensive systems. This is undoubtedly true of any kind of sickness at any age. Among older people waning abilities and numberless discomforts bring about increased self-centeredness or narcissism. When aged persons become preoccupied with self, they reduce their social vision and undergo retrogressive personality changes which render them pathetic, dependent, and irritable. Ours is a child-centered, youth-oriented culture in which age has little status. Those who reach the later years discover that most of the rewards of living have already been experienced.

In our effort to create a sound democratic civilization, we often exaggerate and overinterpret the nature of democracy. Many executives, even the heads of hospitals and mental institutions, boast of creating an atmosphere in which employees and officials meet frequently, dine together in the same cafeterias, and observe few formalities that would separate leaders from followers. I believe this is a mistake. Older persons who have risen to positions of authority deserve a special status and special privileges in compensation for their extra and often arduous responsibilities. After all, none of us enjoys relinquishing youth's freshness and vitality and power to recover. When we must let go of these advantages, should we not at least hold on to the one social advantage of aging, that of status and privilege? The value of these is that they preserve dignity. Aging connotes many losses, and a man, whatever else he must lay aside, should be permitted to retain his dignity. The self-esteem engendered by status is life-preserving. Our Western societies, however, induce a sense of anticlimactic superfluousness in older people, as though they had outlived their usefulness and must accept defeat in intergenerational conflict.

The best social system, which produced the most integrated family life and the sturdiest character fiber, was found in stoic societies, particularly the Roman, during the three-century period before 200 B.C. The stoic family culture preserved in high degree the male patriarchal role of the father and the female maternalistic role of the mother. Children were obedient. Respect of elders was primary. The morality of the children reached an extraordinarily high level. The breakdown of the Roman system followed upon the abdication of the male from his position of responsible leadership, the assumption of that power by the woman, the increase in materialization, and the surrender to hedonism. In the decline and fall of the Roman Empire we can trace a continuous exchange of roles between men and women.

About two centuries ago, when society in the United States was 85 per cent agrarian, the male was the leader of the family. His marriage was rarely romantic; in fact, it was often one of convenience, and women and children were treated as chattels. The industrial revolution, together with the feminist movement, emancipated women and, later on, children. Soon the swing of social reform, like a pendulum, went to the extreme, and males felt themselves eclipsed. With new monetary opportunities, and social equality with men, women progressively assumed a position of dominance.

There can be little doubt that the progressive and continuous exchange of parental roles within families has produced in youngsters an unconscious sense of doubt as to identity, psychosexuality, and feeling of adequacy. Thus an element of unconscious homosexual conflict, which may be viewed as compensatory, sublimatory, and rationalized, has been introduced into the lives of children of both sexes. The exorbitant suppression of children during the latter half of the nineteenth century gave rise to an enormous increase in psychoneurotic disorders. This stimulated a medical response in the form of the development of psychiatry. The sometimes cruel and restrictive method of rearing children had produced encapsulated symptom neuroses. The patient felt that part of him was sick, but that the rest of him was reasonably normal. The psychiatric systems of care proved very effective in dealing with this type of psychological disorder.

But a great change took place in the transition to the twentieth century. Permissiveness was introduced in child discipline. The role exchange in the family between father and mother was intensified. The vast number of immigrants to the United States were young men and women from Europe, who came without their parents and thus had only a tenuous link with their accustomed family atmosphere. Eager to assimilate the new culture, these newcomers rapidly assumed the new principles of family life.

The result of all these factors has been the development of character neuroses in which the entire personality is involved. This is related to the great degree of permissiveness extended to children, the relative absence of the father from the household, the intensification of the mother's leadership role, and the ill-defined role of older people.

Thus today we see three unhappy generations in the United States: (1) the youngest, who are arrogant, prematurely autonomous, anxiety-ridden, and in search of direction; (2) the middle generation, who are bewildered because their authority as parents is paralyzed; and (3) the older generation, who are socially impotent and isolated.

PSYCHOSOCIAL FACTORS

Let us note specifically the psychosocial factors to which the older generation is exposed. Social retirement, as well as eventual economic retirement, is forced upon older people long before their biological condition demands it. The retirement age is of archaic origin. People today are still enjoying robust health in their sixties. The feeling of isolation is based upon several factors:

1. Social mobility. The extent to which younger people move about, partly to follow industry, partly to satisfy a subsurface restlessness, tends to leave older people in constantly changing neighborhoods. Not only do older citizens progressively lose their affectional contacts, but they are forced to feel out of place in the very neighborhood to whose development they may have devoted their entire lives.

2. Youth orientation. The cultural accent on youth leads to neglect of the values of living at other phases of maturation. The aged are set aside by younger people who do not look to their elders as sources of information about living which might be applicable to themselves.

3. Materialism and productivity. There is no longer any question that our society is achievement-oriented. The abstractions of art and related aspects of culture are less valued and less sought after than are physical productivity and the possession of tangible articles. Obviously, in a society thus constituted, those who do not work and who do not seem to be achieving materialistic goals, as is true of the aging, are relegated to the position of second-class citizens.

4. Overvaluation of sexuality and physical attractiveness. There is today abundant evidence that our culture is oriented toward youthful attractiveness and various aspects of sexuality, despite, and in social conflict with, our puritanical heritage. The abstractions of thought, the contributions of the arts, and the deeper philosophical considerations of living are consigned to a far less important position socially than are beauty and sex appeal. The diminution in physical attractiveness in people as they grow older, as well as the tendency of the mature to sublimate most of their instincts, causes the aged to be subtly exiled from the main stream of living.

5. Absence of tradition. Older people tend to perpetuate traditions. Their experiences commonly eventuate in a somewhat conservative attitude, doubtless unconsciously designed for sustaining and perpetuating sound principles. Societies which are more tradition-bound than our own usually foster veneration of the elders. In such cultural settings family life is more closely knit than in our country, and the progeny develop a strong feeling of in-group membership which is extended in folk practices to a broader sense of nationality. Although it is true that tradition interferes to some extent with progress, to a more significant extent it fosters good communications between the generations. In tradition-bound cultures the ego formation of the growing personality is strong and the fiber of character firm. Such factors show marked contrast to the lack of personality development among our people.

Because ours is a youth-oriented, child-centered society, rebelliousness, self-directedness, and what might be termed the inept autonomy of youth, show themselves as a constantly perpetuated effort to destroy tradition and to establish evanescent customs in the guise of progress. The wanton destruction of tradition and the widespread search for novel methods of behavior push the elders aside, precisely because experience has taught them to strive to preserve the established rules of interpersonal relationship.

6. Changes in fashions. The constantly accelerated change in fads and fashions, as espoused by the youth-oriented in our culture, tends to isolate the more stolid oldsters. The latter, much less concerned with change for change's sake alone, are looked upon as obstacles to advance.

The cultural exclusion of older people constitutes social deprivation to which they often respond by losing self-confidence and by feeling useless and lonely; their self-esteem is lowered, their enjoyment reduced, and their insecurity intensified. These tormenting sensations arouse long-suppressed anxiety, terror, and panic. The management of such unpleasant inner experiences encourages overdetermined and extravagant psychologic defenses which become quantitatively and qualitatively pathologic. The cantankerousness, the willfulness, the despotic maneuvering, the insatiability, and the irritability of many older people are based on precisely such defensive manipulations.

Many writers assert that the older person is more serious-minded, more sober, more aware of responsibility, and more capable of assuming obligations than he was earlier. This is only partly true. Older people do not want to be perpetually sober or serious-minded. They, too, like to have fun, enjoy life, and pursue pleasurable activities. There is, however, widespread moroseness among older people. In my estimation, this is undiagnosed and therefore untreated depression, the melancholy found at the outset of most psychological disorders. It must have much to do with decline and breakdown.

PSYCHOLOGICAL FACTORS

People for whom aging is a problem not only react adversely to social pressures and vacuums, but, in addition, manifest certain deep psychic needs. These deep neurotic forces have been present since earliest infancy and childhood, and tend to exacerbate the indispositions of aging. Most commonly found among this group are the following personality syndromes:

1. The sensitive personalities. These are easily hurt, insulted, or outraged, and are particularly self-centered. People in this category are often the victims of overindulgence or overprotection, evidences of subtle rejection early in life.

Their personalities are often characterized by reaction formations against their profound feelings of inadequacy and inferiority.

2. The hostile personalities. Based on unresolved neurotic conflicts and an exorbitant need to be loved, these personalities reveal an incapacity to develop strong interpersonal relationships. Some people in this group have developed a strong undercurrent of resentment against abuses, excessive discipline, and harsh or cruel punitive measures visited upon them in early childhood.

3. The chronically adolescent personalities. These individuals, all too common in our society, reveal an incapacity to identify themselves with the parental image, owing to perpetuation of adolescent rebellion. They have a chronic inability to assume any but a pseudoparental role with a puerile and churlish undercurrent. Individuals who are in rebellion against elders cannot become elders. Their rebellion is accompanied by rebellion against the process of aging.

4. The masochistic personalities. People in this category turn all aggression against themselves. They cannot tolerate their own aggressive and sadistic impulses, and they suffer excessive guilt, chronic depression, and moods of despair. Self-destructive impulses are not uncommon in such individuals.

5. The defensive personalities. These utilize denial, repression, reaction formation, and projection as their main interpersonal currency. They are like prickly burrs, constantly fending off attack, whether real or imagined. Their proclivity for projection often undergoes dereistic transformation into paranoid delusion formation. They avoid anxiety by shifting responsibility and blame to others.

People afflicted in these ways are too busy building and repairing defenses to find the time and energy necessary to penetrate life. Their tendency in earlier years to identify with the predominantly elder-rejecting culture, to perpetuate unresolved hostilities against their elders after earliest psychosexual maturation, and to perpetuate rebellion against their elders and those in authority, now makes them the prime targets of their own attitudes of rejection and hostility, turning anger, aggression, and hatred against themselves to produce depression.

SELF-REJECTION

The atmosphere of passive neglect toward oldsters produces a sequence of psychosocial events: (1) cultural rejection; (2) self-rejection; (3) anxiety, panic, depression; (4) psychophysiologic exhaustion; (5) intrapsychic regression and adaptation in depth; (6) withdrawal of object interest (isolation); (7) phenomena of restitution with enhancement of pathologic defensive maneuvers; and (8) autistic and dereistic internalization and preoccupation.

The sequence of psychological events may be described as follows. At first there are feelings of fatigue, bewilderment, perplexity, and waning alertness, followed by deepening despair and agitation, with confusion and progressive memory impairment. The diminution or loss of mental faculties leads to deep intrapsychic panic which is controlled by the tightening of defense mechanisms. As a result, the aged patient presents the picture of intellectual and emotional deterioration with increased defensiveness and consequent self-isolation.

As the psychic defenses are essentially illusions, they lose some of their effectiveness in a social environment that remains unresponsive and fails to furnish needed emotional nourishment. This loss of effectiveness, in association with biophysiologic decrements, leads to further waning of physical resistances. Therefore increased organic deterioration may be the logical consequence of what began merely as a psychological attitude.

The vicissitudes of aging in our culture belong essentially in the fields of preventive mental treatment and of child psychiatry. The nature of the old man is determined in the years of infancy. This may be paraphrased by the psychological observation that the older a man grows, the more like himself he becomes. But each psychiatric symptom in aging can be understood and treated. Each bit of behavior has meaning. When this meaning is conveyed to the patient, he is armed with new resources and can do battle against his own suffering. It is the obligation of modern psychiatry to equip practitioners to treat the aged appropriately and understandingly, and thus to restore to them some of the dignity and the comfort to which they are entitled.

REFERENCES

1. LINDEN, MAURICE E. Some implications in aging. Am. J. Ortho-psychiat., XXVIII (no. 2):322–328, 1958.
2. LINDEN, MAURICE E., and DOUGLAS COURTNEY. The human life cycle and its interruptions, a psychologic hypothesis. Studies in gerontologic human relations I. Am. J. Psychiat., 109 (no. 12):906–915, 1953.

8   CURRENT TRENDS

IN PSYCHIATRIC

RESEARCH*

BY ALBERT DEUTSCH

IN THEIR ABSORBING BIOGRAPHY of Dr. William Henry Welch, probably the greatest medical statesman in American history, Simon and Thomas Flexner describe the beginnings of the Rockefeller Institute for Medical Research. They tell how the Reverend Frederick T. Gates, a philanthropic adviser of John D. Rockefeller, in 1897 fell upon a copy of Osler's classic *Principles and Practice of Medicine.* The Flexners quote Mr. Gates:

> *"This book not only confirmed my skepticism, but its revelation absolutely astounded and appalled me. . . . I found, for illustration, that our best medical practice did not, and did not pretend to, cure more than four or five diseases. That is, medicine had at that time specifics for about as many diseases as there are fingers on one hand. . . .*

> *"To the layman student like me, demanding cures and specifics, he (Osler) had no word of comfort whatever. In fact, I saw clearly from the work of this able and honest man that medicine had, with the few exceptions above mentioned, no cures, and that about all that medicine up to 1897 could do was to nurse the patients and alleviate in some degree the suffering. . . .*
>
> *"When I laid down this book I had begun to realize how woefully neglected in all civilized countries, and perhaps most of all in this country, had been the scientific study of medicine. . . ."*

The rest is medical history: Mr. Gates transmitted his sense of shock to Mr. Rockefeller, who nodded his head, and then the statesmanship of Dr. Welch and other medical greats was enlisted to organize the great research center.

If the good Mr. Gates was "astounded and appalled" by the paucity of cures in general medicine at the turn of the century, what would his reaction be to the comparable state of psychiatric therapeutics today? What great changes have been wrought in medicine in the first six decades of the twentieth century? The Rockefeller Institute, the first great American center devoted primarily to medical research, concentrated its efforts mainly against the great challenge of the time —infectious diseases. Today, most of the infectious diseases have been brought under control by advancing medical science. The great challenge to contemporary medical science comprises the chronic ailments, with mental ills in the forefront.

Psychiatry in Medicine

Like Mr. Gates, I am a layman in medicine. Like him, my interest in research was spurred by the revelation of inadequacies in the therapeutic field. Not by reading a single classic, but by years of study—first as a historian, then as a journalist—of the treatment, nontreatment, and maltreatment of the mentally ill in the United States, I became convinced that the fuller application of extant psychiatric knowledge was not enough. I joined the growing body of people who believe that the next great push in the mental health field must be in the direction of gaining new knowledge through scientific research. About three years ago I set out upon a journalistic survey which took me to scores of mental health research centers across the country. I have interviewed more than a hundred investigators and pored over hundreds of research papers and reports. It has been a rich and rewarding experience for me personally. In this paper I can do no more than select, from the welter of material, a series of impressions of what I have seen, heard, and—I hope—digested in my rounds.

Perhaps the single outstanding characteristic of this research enterprise is the almost explosive expansion of the past decade or so. A second distinction is a rise of quality, though not quite at the same tempo as the increase in research activity. A third is the almost bewildering diversity of projects and programs, together with the broad range of scientific personnel engaged in them. A fourth is the persistence of grave shortages of high-grade investigative manpower, paradoxically but understandably growing more serious as the total research enterprise steadily expands.

When I started to prepare my history of American psychiatric treatment in 1934, mental hygiene specialists were still aglow with the thrill of the announcement made the previous year that the Scottish Rite Masons, Northern Jurisdiction, had voted an annual fund of $40,000 for research in schizophrenia. So seriously impoverished was the psychiatric research effort at the time that some enthusiasts headily predicted that the most devastating of all mental diseases would soon be conquered by the sheer thrust of this financial avalanche.

In 1936 the National Committee for Mental Hygiene embarked on a survey of research in American tax-supported psychiatric institutions. Its report, published in 1938, revealed that of 273 psychiatric hospitals and institutes covered, only 20—less than 8 per cent—had any research in progress, and 32 more were listed as being capable of conducting research if they had the staff, money, and motivation. With few exceptions, the ongoing research was judged to be of poor quality.

The situation had improved but little by the end of World War II, and in some areas it had regressed. But the lessons of that war—in manifold, complex, and sometimes contradictory ways, which have often been cited in the literature and need no retelling here—provided a tremendous stimulus to scientific research in general, to medical research, and to the sciences of human behavior, especially of the mind in health and illness.

The creation by congressional act in 1946 of the National Institute of Mental Health within the U.S. Public Health Service proved to be the greatest single spur to psychiatric research in our history. It marked the beginning of a proliferation of investigative activities which is truly breathtaking. Philip Sapir, in a recent study, notes that the number of research projects and programs throughout the country supported by NIMH has multiplied thirtyfold since 1948, and that the funds expended by NIMH have multiplied sixtyfold. In the fiscal year 1961, NIMH alone is spending more than $50,000,000 for intramural and extramural research and for the training of investigators. This sum represents more than half the estimated mental health research financing from all sources in the United States. Our federal agencies, including the Veterans Administration, the Department of Defense, and the National Science Foundation, expend about $9,000,000 more for behavioral research. State government funds used for this purpose total about $14,000,000 annually. Dr. Jeanne Brand, who has just completed a survey of American private foundations making grants for mental health research, lists nearly 122 such national agencies granting a total of about $4,000,000 a year.

Dr. William Soskin, in a forthcoming monograph of the Joint Commission on Mental Illness and Health, reports: "At the peak period of interest in the development of the new market for psychotherapeutic drugs the pharmaceutical industry in 1957–1959 invested about $12,000,000 per year on psychotherapeutic drugs, about $10,000,000 of which was for research within the industry's own laboratories and the remainder for drug testing and free research grants to investigators in universities, state hospitals and similar settings." This figure seems overoptimistic to me, but it is all we have. There is no national estimate at all for direct university expenditures on mental health research or for grants made for this purpose by private individuals or industrial concerns. Because of the broadly blurred boundaries and widely varying definitions of "mental health," even the estimates we have at hand are of the roughest character. It would seem, then, that these rough estimates, gleaned from several sources, indicate a total annual expenditure of about $90,000,000 for mental health research in the United States. That is still only a modest fraction of what goes into missile research alone, and far below the optimum in wise investment in the emotional stability of mankind at home and abroad. But it would loom unbelievably stupendous to the "mental healthers" of a quarter-century ago who thrilled to the news of a $40,000 windfall.

Indeed, a bare two decades ago, scientific investigators in the mental health field were a pitifully small, widely scattered, financially malnourished band, ignored and often despised by the scientific community and the public at large. Today they are a rapidly growing legion, working with far better tools, with better-prepared skills, and with greatly enhanced knowledge in more encouraging environments, asking sharper questions, and anticipating sounder payoffs. One is awed by the breadth, the intensity, and the variety of the research, and by the diversity of the scientists engaged in it.

On many fronts and with many maneuvers, the research assault on mental illness is being waged by psychiatrists, psychologists, biochemists, biostatisticians, pharmacologists, neurologists, geneticists, physiologists, anatomists, pathologists, sociologists, anthropologists, biophysicists, and a host of hyphenated specialists covering a wide range of the scientific fellowship. In truth, it becomes increasingly awkward to continue to designate as "psychiatric research" a field in which, as Dr. Soskin points out in his unpublished study, psychiatrists represent less than one-tenth of the professional investigators in the field. "Mental health research" is itself a clumsy and ambiguous term, but it seems more descriptive of the total enterprise at this point.

One of the most encouraging developments in recent years has been the active enlistment of distinguished "outside" scientists, responding to what is probably the greatest challenge not only to medical science but to all science—the study of human behavior. Along with this heartening development, one sees increasing numbers of younger men of quality, standing on the threshold of a scientific career, choose research in mental health as a lifework in preference to other areas of investigation.

Those engaged in this great enterprise work in a kaleidoscopic variety of settings. Sometimes they work singly, sometimes in combination. Some work on a grand design, stretching over the whole reach of mental health, even to unitary concepts of human behavior. Others work on a microscopic part of the whole problem, proving the mysteries of a single cell or the function of a specific neuron. Some work with animals, some with humans, in laboratories or in clinical settings. Some are concerned with organic approaches, others with psychological hypotheses, and still others with both. The molecule, the individual organism, the family constellation, the social and cultural environment—all these are legitimate foci of mental health research.

Here a physiologist, with pinpoint precision, plants an electrode in a minute spot of the brain of a human, a monkey, or a rat, to gather information on specific centers or pathways of mental and emotional behavior. There an investigator works with infinite patience to contribute some speck of information on the anatomical or chemical cartography of a particular area of the central nervous system. Here an anthropologist lives for weeks in the home of a schizophrenic patient, studying family interaction in a natural setting. There a group of social scientists survey a whole community to find clues to the ecology of the epidemiology of mental disorder.

A pharmacologist works on a new drug. A daring psychoanalyst permits the long-cherished sanctity of his couch to be violated by the presence of scientific observers bent on evaluating the therapeutic process of his discipline, or even to have the patient-analyst transaction televised for research purposes. A biochemist minutely studies the blood or the urine of a schizophrenic patient for possible clues to the etiology or process of the disease. A biophysicist uses the latest products of nuclear reactors as new weapons in the fight against an age-old scourge. A team of investigators studies child victims of phenylketonuria for leads to a possible molecular basis for all mental diseases. Researchers in a nationwide network of mental hospitals conduct a coöperative study in the evaluation of tranquilizing and other new drugs. A young career investigator spends many sleepless hours observing and making minute recordings of the behavior of a newborn babe. Social scientists around the world systematically gather and exchange new information on the transcultural aspects of mental illness.

The quality of this expanding research effort is not uniformly good, by any means. It ranges from excellent through mediocre to very poor. But the general level is steadily improving. It adds up to an ever-growing bank of scientific data which must eventually lead to the goals of reducing mental illness and reaching toward optimum mental health.

The student of current trends is greatly encouraged by the development of scientific sophistication in a field notorious for its fumbling generalizations, its faddism in hasty acceptance of unproved theory and ill-tried therapies, its deficiency of self-criticism, its overload of rigid and mutually contradictory dogmatisms, its use of defensive invective in place of solid data. There is a distinct trend toward critical evaluation of theories and therapies long taken for granted, toward less status-seeking at the expense of truth-seeking, toward more active concern for sharper definition and greater specificity.

There has been much discussion, pro and con, about the trend toward interdisciplinary or multidisciplinary psychiatric research. It seems to me that this controversy is largely academic. In the light of the growing multiplicity and complexity of new research instruments, and of the rapid proliferation of scientific knowledge, it is futile to argue whether we should have more or less interdisciplinary research. The trend can no longer be viewed as being desirable or undesirable; it is necessary and inevitable. There remains plenty of room and plenty of opportunity for the unreconstructed "loner" to operate fruitfully.

As a journalistic observer, I am intrigued by the rich variations in personality among the researchers I have interviewed. It is impossible to fit them into a pat composite "profile" of the scientist. I asked two outstanding men, separately, what motivated them to go into mental health research. One replied: "Curosity, that's all. My object is no nobler than that." The other answered: "I want to help alleviate the sufferings of my fellow men, and to help give greater dignity to the race." Both are first-rate scientists and fine human beings.

One of the distinct benefits of the newer knowledge emanating from behavioral research is the searchlight it throws on the vast swamplands of ignorance in which psychiatry still wallows. The inescapable awareness of this unexplored ignorance compels a more becoming and a more realistic modesty. One perceives a marked reduction in dogmatic assertions among the several schools and approaches, less sectarian contention, greater self-searching, more opening of the mind to the ideological views of others. With it comes a weakening of the old dichotomies—heredity versus environment, laboratory versus clinic, organic versus psychological.

To be sure, one still hears a dogmatic organicist mumble: "If it can't be measured, it isn't science." Or a dogmatic psychoanalyst may ask querulously: "What can you learn about the human psyche from watching rats jump? What can statistics tell you about the unconscious?" I recall, at the height of the overoptimistic wave that followed the introduction of tranquilizing drugs, an inveterate analyst-baiter who told me: "Freud is dead. Now it's official. Even the psychoanalysts must recognize that they've had their day. Psychiatry has at last shaken off the yoke of Freudian enslavement. From now on, it's biochemistry, pure and simple."

Had that man been a sober student of psychiatric history, he would have been rendered more modest by contemplation of the long, long list of chemical "cures" that cometed across the psychiatric horizon, creating public sensation, only to pass into oblivion. There was the morphine "cure" for mental illness, the bromides, the barbiturates, even aspirin, to mention only a few. Indeed, organic approaches dominated psychiatric research throughout the nineteenth century; the so-called psychological or Freudian dominance is of relatively recent vintage. Beyond the biochemical, the student of psychiatric history could point to an almost limitless list of organic "cures" touted as great breakthroughs in therapy before wide use revealed them as miserable failures. In the latter part of the eighteenth century, mental patients were bled white, sometimes unto death, here and abroad, on the widely held theory that madness was caused by bad blood. Others were stuffed with noxious pills and purgatives. One need only note, in passing, the series of surgical procedures that arose as sensational cures for mental disease before their destructive futility was revealed. Among the more recent were the mass operations on mental patients resulting from enthusiastic adherence to the "focal infection" theory, and the indiscriminate mass lobotomies of later date. Returning to the biochemical angle, one recalls vividly the recent excitement over ceruloplasmin, and the melancholy post-mortem in Seymour Kety's classic review of current biochemical theories of schizophrenia, published in *Science:* "The rise and fall of ceruloplasmin as a biochemical factor significantly related to schizophrenia is one of the briefest if not the most enlightening chapter in the history of biological psychiatry." In that same paper, you will recall, Kety, a physiologist who stands in the forefront of contemporary psychiatric research, concluded his brilliant analysis with this observation: "Although the evidence for the great importance of genetic and therefore biological factors in the etiology of many or all of the schizophrenics is quite compelling, the signposts pointing the way to their discovery are at present quite blurred and, to me at least, illegible."

As for psychoanalysis, it seemed for a time that Freudians would demonstrate, through their attitude, the validity of Thomas Huxley's observation that it is the fate of new truths to begin as heresies and end as superstitions. Not that the stigma of dogmatism could ever be justifiably stamped on the whole of the Freudian fellowship or even on a considerable part of it, but there have been enough rigid sectarians, often articulate and in positions of influential leadership, who invited the wholesale application. Freud, despite his contests with personal friends and followers, remained imbued with scientific skepticism to the end, testing and retesting his hypotheses, continually modifying his theories to fit newly discovered data. Many leading analysts, beginning with the master himself, had impressive training in neuroanatomy and neurology before they entered their ultimate discipline. Yet one imagines there was many an occasion when Freud, paraphrasing Marx, must have muttered: "God save me from the Freudians."

One cannot deny that forbidding walls still stand between those who give narrow allegiance to either the psychological or the somatic approach. One cannot deny occasional encounters with researchers who behave more like sectarians or cultists than like scientists. But the old walls are being breached in strategic places, and one finds a far greater leavening of the traditional antagonisms, especially among the younger men, correlated with a growing mutual tolerance and respect and a trend toward merging. It is no longer rare to see a neurophysiologist working side by side with a psychoanalyst in a common endeavor, as instanced by the collaboration of William DeMent and Charles Fisher in dream study, or of John Benjamin and his closely knit interdisciplinary staff in the longitudinal study of child development. Often training in several disciplines is merged in one investigator, as witnessed by the work of Arthur Mirsky in Pittsburgh and of Jules Masserman in Chicago.

Even the idioms of the different disciplines are interchanged easily—sometimes too easily. I recall interviewing one of Dr. Magoun's brilliant young investigators, a psychologist conducting brain self-stimulation experiments and seemingly on the track of what was then intriguingly called "the pleasure centers of the brain." I asked what he was about, and he replied: "I'm trying to locate the site of the id." A neurophysiologist doing similar work suddenly interrupted an interview and rushed out of the laboratory exclaiming, "I almost forgot. I simply musn't be late for my analytic hour." Not long ago I even heard a research neurologist mention the tabooed term "human mind" without blushing.

Those who intimate that this field of investigation is already saturated and overfinanced simply do not know what they are talking about. Recently I had occasion to visit a team of investigators who are making significant contributions to behavioral science. They are housed in an appalling scientific slum, with inadequate space and inadequate equipment, and so crowded that the scientists are developing stooped shoulders because they have no room to stand straight. The director, a gifted and dedicated scientist, remarked, "We don't mind it so much, but our experimental animals do."

There are still large gaps in the research effort, great problems that are barely touched. One need only mention the grossly neglected field of research in mental retardation. Here hope comes from a surprising quarter. Several years ago, when the successful mass demonstration of the Salk vaccine was announced, a psychiatrist friend of mine recalled how President Roosevelt's physical affliction had inspired the antipolio movement, and he added, dryly, "Let's hope we get a president who goes crazy; then we may get the wherewithal to conquer mental disease." Well, we have a president who is robustly sane but who, most regrettably from the personal and the family viewpoint, but fortunately from the standpoint of human betterment, has a mentally retarded sister. The President's family, very sensibly, has never tried to shield this fact from the public eye; indeed, the Kennedy family foundation has contributed generously to the study and treatment of mental retardation. The recent presidential creation of the Child Development Center at the National Institute of Health is regarded with concern by many as cutting into the territory of NIMH. Nonetheless, we may now expect a considerable increase in federal aid to research in mental retardation.

The most desperate need of all, of course, is trained manpower for psychiatric research. The difficulty of narrowing the gap between research manpower needs and resources, especially in the higher echelons, is perhaps the greatest single handicap to optimum development of the research endeavor. At every point the competition for gifted young people is keen, and is growing keener. The solution of the manpower dilemma, in the final analysis, involves profound changes in our entire value system—changes that are evolving now, but not fast enough to catch up with the need.

I have presented, in this paper, a very sketchy, highly impressionistic panorama. I should have liked, not only to mention, but also to discuss in some depth, such problems as the significance of federal hegemony in research financing, the upsurge of research activity in mental hospital systems, and human relations in multidisciplinary research, as well as factors in organization and administration. Perhaps it is fitting for me, a laymen, to conclude with a few brief observations on the role of the public in the research effort. It is, after all, largely the dramatic turnabout in public attitudes toward research—from distrust and disinterest to admiration, enthusiasm, and even awe—which has made possible the advances of recent years.

The layman, naturally enough, is most interested in those fruits of research which have immediate application, especially in cures. A great deal of public interest is generated by the announcement of a discovery of a new therapeutic tool. Sometimes, as in the recent introduction of tranquilizing drugs, an overenthusiastic claim leads to sensational stories of "miracle cures." Such stories tend to enliven public interest and to stimulate public support of psychiatric research. But there is always the danger of a cynical apathy inherent in repeated disillusionments.

It seems to me that there is too much talk of breakthroughs on the therapeutic front, even among psychiatrists. This exaggeration of research accomplishments gives the false impression that the big one-shot cure for mental disease is just around the corner. The public must be made more aware of the very great problems that await solution. It must be better informed of the years and years of painstaking basic research behind such spectacular developments as the atomic bomb, the Salk vaccine, and most new therapies that burst seemingly full-blown before the public eye.

The ultimate answers to the basic problems of human behavior in health and illness are still a long way in the future. The fundamental concern of contemporary psychiatric research seems to be in developing the appropriate questions.

9

THE PSYCHIATRIC

ROLE OF THE GENERAL

PRACTITIONER

BY ERIC D. WITTKOWER, M.D.

(with the assistance of William Stauble, M.D.)

INTEREST IN THE psychiatric role of the general practitioner has recently deepened, principally because (1) progressive urbanization and the ensuing anonymity of town life confine patient-doctor contacts to mere professional relationships, and prevent doctors from seeing patients and their families in action and interaction; (2) rapid advances in psychiatry, with their reflection in the daily press and other mass media, have aroused interest in psychiatry and have increased public demand for psychiatric service; (3) from 10 to 50 per cent of the clientele of general practitioners consists of patients suffering from emotional problems; (4) the fragmentation of the medical profession resulting from increasing specialization has revealed a need for an all-embracing, integrated approach by a single person; and (5) the advent of various new drugs, such as the antibiotics, has somewhat depersonalized the doctor-patient relationship.

Unfortunately, or perhaps fortunately, the one-ill, one-pill, one-bill doctor is a thing of the past. It has been sarcastically, and unfairly, stated that the general practitioner has become the middleman between the patient and the diagnostic laboratories, or between the patient and the pharmaceutical industry. This is, of course, a gross exaggeration, but there is consensus on the urgent need for the medical profession as a whole to take into account emotional factors in the pathogenesis of disease and to deal with the mental state of sufferers irrespective of the nature of their illness.

The term "psychiatric" in the title of this paper refers to psychological problems rather than to psychological abnormalities. It is obviously debatable whether the psychiatric role is regarded by the average practitioner as of major importance. The human factor in disease concerns doctor and patient alike, and therefore it seems logical to divide this discussion into three parts: one dealing with the patient, the second with the doctor, and the third with the doctor-patient relationship. The main emphasis is placed on the psychological problems of physically sick patients and the problems of the doctors attending them.

PSYCHOLOGICAL PROBLEMS

The psychiatric role of the general practitioner covers a wide field. Theoretically and ideally, it encompasses (1) appraisal of the degree of organic and/or psychological involvement in a given patient; (2) appraisal of the relevance of emotional factors to the etiology of the disease and its exacerbations; (3) appraisal of the secondary effects of the disease on cerebral function; (4) appraisal of the patient's premorbid personality; (5) understanding of the psychology of the sick person; (6) understanding of the patient's responses to therapeutic procedures; and (7) awareness of the interactions that take place between patient and doctor.

The complexity of the problem is revealed by the work of Reiser and his associates on heart disease (11). They point out that significant life events or situations (including the diagnosis of heart disease itself), which are attended by anxiety and emotional tensions, may well contribute to the development of congestive failure, cardiac arrhythmia, and myocardial ischemia; that chronic cerebral anoxia or repeated acute episodes, as in the Stokes-Adams syndrome, may accelerate vascular degenerative brain disease and thus contribute to the development of degenerative organic dementias; that maladjustment to the handicaps imposed by the heart disease, combined with psychological mismanagement by the treating physician, may lead to unwarranted invalidism, harmful overactivity, or other modes of behavior which are against the best interests of the patient.

Obviously it is neither necessary nor possible for the busy general practitioner, owing to the lack of time or of training, to cover all these points; but it is equally obvious that diagnostic and therapeutic neglect may lead to costly and often unnecessary laboratory procedures, to the development of iatrogenic symptoms, and not infrequently to polysurgery, before the patient lands at the doorstep of a psychiatrist, or of a quack. Moreover, it is probably agreed that, within limits, the success of the practitioner, therapeutically and financially, depends less upon his scientific knowledge than upon his manner with patients. Certainly, in order to handle patients successfully, he must understand their psychology.

THE PATIENT

In common parlance, we *feel* sick, but we do not *feel* healthy. A state of health is taken for granted, and only disturbances in health are noticed by the affected person and by others. We know that we may become ill and that we must some day die, but neither illness nor death is a matter of undue concern for the physically healthy and emotionally well-adjusted individual. Denial of the contingency of illness and of death is a necessity of normal functioning.

Initial stages. The first response to "not feeling well" is often vague and ill defined. During this early "unorganized period of illness" (2), which may last for a few minutes or a few years, a patient not infrequently loses interest in his environment, and this may indeed be the only evidence of the existing or approaching illness. As Stainbrook puts it, "The individual who is feeling ill may not know very clearly how to define his distress either physiologically or psychologically. He may, under certain circumstances, take a covert sick role in which he alone is involved. . . . Many such patients, before occupying an overt sick role, privately accept themselves as sick and use their self-validated sick role as a way of rationalizing inadequacies of self-realization, achievement and participation" (13). To ward off the threat to himself arising from the still dormant illness, a person at this stage is apt to use the ego defense mechanism of denial, attributing his malaise to trivial causes. As this defense mechanism fails to function under the impact of mounting stimuli from within, the patient's ego may suffer anxiety, although he is still unable to define its source. Thus feelings of anxiety, as the signal of an approaching organic illness, may be the one and only symptom the patient is aware of at the time he seeks medical help.

The importance of denial as a factor in delaying initial patient-doctor contact cannot be overemphasized. Our own research on patients suffering from cancer and tuberculosis has shown that patients, even in the face of incontrovertible evidence of the existence of illness, avoid seeking medical help rather than learn the unpalatable truth. Ignorance, it is said, means bliss; denial of illness is, unconsciously, conviction of its absence. The delay in initial patient-doctor contact in cases of serious disease is to some extent unrelated to knowledge, because doctors and nurses are just as guilty of it as others, and even Freud "denied" the existence of his cancer for some time before he decided to consult a doctor.

Denial in this context is a refutation of the existence of something known to exist. This "something" may be a serious, allegedly incurable disease, or it may be anything else, and the refutation may be total or partial. Typically, one of our cancer patients, unconsciously striking a compromise with himself, presented himself with a common cold, apparently oblivious of unmistakable signs of cancer. Similarly, one of Hollender's patients complained of pelvic pain when what she actually wanted was help with her problem of sexual frigidity. In another patient, the presenting symptom of hemorrhoids, which required operation, concealed his concern about an impending schizophrenic breakdown (5).

Diagnosis. At the time when a patient presents himself to a doctor, he obviously does not want to hear that there is something dreadfully wrong which may prove fatal. He hopes to be told, often despite clear evidence to the contrary, that there is nothing to worry about and that he will shortly be well. When his erroneous belief, which amounts to a partial denial, is shattered by confrontation with a serious diagnosis, he may be thrown into anxiety and despair which are founded not only on realistic considerations but also on the culturally ascribed significance of the diagnosed illness, on common beliefs, and on its personally experienced symbolic meaning. This breach in his psychological defense system, which to some extent may be desirable for the acceptance of his sick role, is closed again if the patient meets the threat of potential annihilation and symbolic castration by rejecting the diagnosis and defiantly disregarding the doctor's instructions. Some patients experience a sense of relief even on being confronted with a serious diagnosis, just as a phobia is preferable to morbid anxiety without clearly defined content. Others, consciously or unconsciously, welcome illness as an escape from life with which they are unable to cope, or as a well-deserved punishment. But, more often than not, patients who profess to be glad they will at long last have a much-needed rest, deceive themselves and use either a manic defense or the mechanism of rationalization.

The illness. As previously noted, illness leads to a withdrawal of interest from the environment. The withdrawn interest is invested in the imperiled self. If my house is on fire, my immediate concern does not go much farther than my neighbor's property; and if I am ill, my ill-health is my main concern. Hence, almost invariably, seriously and chronically ill persons become self-centered. The degree of this disease narcissism depends on four main factors: (1) the amount of constitutional narcissism, (2) the real or imagined seriousness of the illness, (3) the nature of the illness, and (4) the organ affected. Ferenczi, in his classical paper on disease and patho-neurosis, points out that disfiguring diseases, diseases of and injuries to the eyes, and diseases of the genitalia evoke, more than others, a regression to disease narcissism (4). He suggests, for instance, that puerperal psychoses should be attributed to the unavoidable injury to the central erotogenic zone at parturition rather than to infection.

It appears that, in many cases, the libido which is withdrawn from the outer world is not directed toward the whole ego but, magnetlike, to the diseased or injured organ. As a result of this local accumulation of libido, symptoms may come into evidence which are not directly related to the structural lesion: vague shifting pains in the cardiac region in persons who know they suffer from cardiac disease; eyestrain, blurring of sight, photophobia, and night blindness in persons who have lost vision in one eye; or pruritus vulvae in connection with prolonged gynecological disorders. Symptoms may also persist after the actual disease has ceased to exist, as coughing after whooping cough.

Although illness leads to a traumatic narcissism, it also leads at the same time to a growing demand for narcissistic supplies. Illness invariably lowers oneself in the esteem of others and in one's own self-esteem. Yesterday one was a fully functioning person on equal standing with other members of the working community; today one is a patient, only a patient, or only another case among many. Concomitantly there is a devaluation in self-esteem. Health is highly prized, and ill-health, with its incapacitating effects, may be experienced as defaulting. It is hardly surprising that persons who are suffering from serious or prolonged illness, or who are permanently disabled, are often seriously depressed and seek evidence that they are loved, still loved, or still lovable. This state of depression and this need for affection, an inevitable result of illness, may be related to loss in various spheres, to frustration, to helplessness, and to a real or imagined threat to life. But it may also arise from feelings of guilt, though there is no justification for feeling guilty at being ill. A person who feels guilty at being ill—or, more specifically, at letting his family down by reason of his illness—reveals that he is vaguely aware of a concealed aggressive aim or purpose in his illness which he cannot tolerate. For instance, a person whose illness is motivated by conflicts over ambivalence, or whose conflicts over ambivalence have been intensified by his illness, is likely to be in greater need of affection than others because he is afraid of being found out and because he wants to be reassured that this has not happened yet.

Another way of dealing with loss is by replacement in fantasy. Anybody who has had experience with chronically sick and permanently disabled persons must have noted that they spend hours in reverie, daydreaming about what they could have done, what they might have done, and what they will do (although they never will).

Closely related to withdrawal of interest and fantasy-building is regression, a partial return to and retreat into the past, with revival and emergence of infantile forms of behavior. There is plenty of phenomenological evidence of this psychological process, such as the curling up of many patients in pain in a fetal position; the "naughtiness" of the sick, culminating in childish temper tantrums; and the wish of certain patients to be fed, washed, rubbed, and helped beyond the stage when these attentions are still necessary. Known to all of us, too, is the suggestibility of many sick persons and their blind belief in the doctor's magic powers.

This move into regression is, of course, facilitated and fostered in varying degrees by those who attend the sick. Freed from the burden of his social obligations, and exempted from responsibility for his state of being helpless, the sick person is supposed to surrender to the care of those who know best what is good for him. Indulgence is shown for his little foibles, and restrictions are imposed on him which he is supposed to accept in a docile manner. Everyday experience shows that a person's value goes up if there is a likelihood or risk of his departure. Friends or relatives, whether they have been truly attached to or have harbored hostile feelings toward a person, experience concern when that person is seriously ill, and show by word and by deed how deep their concern may be. By so doing they feed the patient's egocentricity and encourage a move into regression.

What is the function of regression in patients suffering from organic illness? Several answers may be given to this question. Regression may be understood as a defensive withdrawal from a situation with which the patient's ego is unable to cope, as a revival of the stage of development where the parents were always present to protect him in his helplessness (with the omniscient and omnipotent doctor taking over their role); or it may be regarded as an unconscious attempt at literally making a new start. A recuperating patient often feels "newborn," and sometimes says, quite seriously, that the physician has given him a "new life" (9).

THE DOCTOR

Persons who take up the medical profession do so for sociological, economic, and psychological reasons. The profession holds honor and prestige; it provides an adequate income; and it enables its practitioners to feel the gratification that comes from helping the sick and the needy and from relieving pain and suffering. Yet behind these conscious motivations may be unconscious motivations which can be traced back to infantile instinctual drives and conflicts arising from them (7, 8, 9, 12). If incompletely resolved, these conflicts may give rise to serious difficulties in professional performance.

Identification. Identification with a father who sets a shining example as a doctor and perhaps advises his son to follow in his footsteps may be quite conscious, and, if success-fully carried off, may, indeed, in deep layers of the mind, con-stitute a successful solution of the Oedipus complex. But, hidden behind the endeavor to emulate the father, and going beyond it, may be the conscious or unconscious wish to out-shine him, to humiliate him, to annihilate him, and perhaps to curry favor with the mother. Simmel and Nunberg (12, 9) have pointed out that children often alternate between the father-and-mother game and the doctor game, and that at least one determinant of the doctor game is the wish to take over the much-desired role of the father. Alternatively, the choice of the medical profession may be prompted by identi-fication with the mother, whose tenderness and whose com-fort-giving and pain-relieving capacities the would-be doctor at one time admired and enjoyed. Or the object of identifica-tion may be neither father nor mother but the much-revered figure of a family doctor, who helped the person aspiring to be a doctor himself, as well as seriously ill members of his family. The aim then in becoming a doctor is a savior fantasy regard-ing primarily the family and, ultimately, suffering mankind in general.

Omnipotence. The doctor game serves another pur-pose. By playing it the little boy repeats in an active fashion a previous frightening, passive experience. It therefore allows him to overcome fear of the father (by identification with the aggressor); to acquire power over his mother; and, beyond this, in fantasy to become omiscient, as at one time he believed his parents to be. Should such a person later become a doctor, the belief in his omniscience and omnipotence, which may have played a part in his choice of a profession, is reinforced by the power that doctors, thanks to their knowledge and assigned role, wield in society. This power, which amounts at times to power over life and death, may be put to good use. But if infantile omnipotence fantasies have not been adequately curbed by reality testing, the doctor may become pompous, bumptious, and conceited, or, worse than this, blind to his own limitations. He may be tempted to accept and to undertake professional tasks that should have been handed over to colleagues of greater knowledge and skill.

Narcissism. Closely related to persistence of magical omnipotence fantasies is the persistence of undue narcissism. A doctor who puts out his plate naturally hopes that patients will flock to his office, that he will make a name for himself, and that he will earn a comfortable living. All of us are pleased if at times we make a correct diagnosis or succeed in treatment where others have failed. If this pride in achievement, however, is founded on vanity, then success for the sake of success becomes a primary objective, and the patient's well-being is disregarded.

Curiosity. Another derivative of infantile instinctual drives is the doctor's curiosity. Again reference may be made to the doctor's game during which children often explore one another, especially their genitals. This early curiosity, which is prohibited and may lead to punishment, may be successfully sublimated as an element in the performance of the doctor's professional duties. If, however, owing to faulty psychosexual development, adequate sublimation has failed to materialize, the doctor may be seriously disturbed in carrying out his duties. Conversely, oversevere taboos on curiosity may constitute a handicap in the doctor's diagnostic interests and, specifically, if camouflaged as scientific objectivity, may prevent him from probing into a patient's emotional and sexual life.

Sadism. Finally, psychoanalytical observations have shown that the doctor's compassion and healing intent—both major factors in the choice of the medical profession—are based on guilt over aggressive and destructive impulses. The very term "compassion" implies guilt-motivated identification with the sufferer.

Three vicissitudes of the original impulse of aggressiveness may occur: (1) it may be successfully sublimated, (2) sublimation may be incomplete, and (3) the impulse may be unduly inhibited or reparative needs may prevail. It is obvious that the medical practitioner, in order to be effective, requires a harmonious balance between sublimated aggressiveness and "sublimated utilization of impulses of reparation" (7). Any disturbance of this balance leads to malfunction if not to malpractice.

Incomplete control over aggressive impulses on the part of the doctor may lead to grievous physical or mental harm to the patient. Conversely, if feelings of guilt and reparative needs arising from them prevail in the doctor, he is not only likely to exert himself for his patient in a self-sacrificing and frequently masochistic manner, but he is also running the risk of being too active or too passive. "Both these attitudes," Nunberg has pointed out, "are unconsciously intended to relieve the physician's conscience rather than to cure his patients."

THE DOCTOR-PATIENT RELATIONSHIP

According to Szasz and Hollender (5), there are three models of doctor-patient relationship: (1) activity-passivity, (2) guidance-coöperation, and (3) mutual participation.

Activity-passivity. An example of this model is the handling of a comatose patient. In this case (1) no interaction between the partners of the unit is possible; (2) the doctor is in complete control; (3) it would be an encumbrance for him to identify with the patient; and (4) it would distort his judgment and could interfere with his action if he were to respond emotionally to the patient's suffering. Irrespective of his conscious or unconscious motivations in dealing with the patient, all that matters is the doctor's technical competence. There is similarity here between the patient and a helpless infant, and between the physician and a parent.

Guidance-coöperation. The second model is exemplified by the handling of a patient suffering from an acute infectious disease. This differs from the previous model insofar as the patient is seeking not only the doctor's technical skill but also his help and advice, and insofar as the success of measures prescribed depends to a large extent on the patient's coöperation. Here the doctor is placed in a position of power.

He knows best what is good for the patient, whereas the patient is expected to carry out instructions and is apt to revere the doctor as the healer. This model has its prototype in the relationship of a parent and his adolescent child.

Mutual participation. In the third model, applicable to some chronic diseases and to the process of psychoanalysis, the participants in interaction have approximately equal power, are mutually interdependent, and engage in activity satisfying to both. The aim of the doctor in this type of interaction is to help the patient to help himself, and the aim of the patient is to take care of himself, as indeed he may well do, for instance, in the case of diabetes mellitus. This doctor-patient relationship is an adult-adult relationship.

Of the three models described, the first requires no empathy (merely technical skill), the second requires some empathy, and the third requires a great deal of empathy. The term empathy signifies the capacity to feel into, that is, to appreciate another person's feelings without joining them. It differs from sympathy insofar as the latter means entering into the feelings of another person and becoming affected as he is. Because sympathy (which amounts to emotional involvement in the suffering of a patient) may constitute an unbearable strain, the doctor may swing over defensively to the extreme opposite and adopt a detached, impersonal, so-called scientific attitude toward the patient.

All three models may be present in different stages of the same treatment. Guidance-coöperation, by far the most common model of doctor-patient interaction, requires some elaboration.

In the face of a situation with which he cannot cope alone, the patient turns to the doctor, as at one time he turned to his parents, with the hope that the doctor can repair what perhaps cannot be repaired. Or perhaps he operates on two planes: an adult plane on which he realizes the doctor's limitations, and a childlike regressive plane on which he endows the doctor with superhuman magic qualities. In other words, because of his concern regarding himself, and perhaps because of doubts in the doctor's ability to help him, he magnifies the doctor's powers. If one's fantasy enlarges a person to more than life-size and endows him with a giant's strength, one feels small, helpless, and fearful. Thus confidence in and admiration for the doctor are mingled with distrust and fear, on irrational as well as on rational grounds.

How does a doctor respond to this situation? He may realize the motives behind a patient's fantasy and deal with it accordingly. If the fantasy is unrecognized by the doctor, he accepts it as truth and uses it to feed his self-adulation. "If my patients believe that I am wonderful," he seems to argue, "there must be some justification for their assumption." Doctors may bask in the glory of their successes but, as we all know, the medical profession is beset with many anxieties and is full of risks, failures, and disappointments. Very few doctors can tolerate lack of success in therapy or hostility from their patients. It is no wonder that neurotic patients are unpopular in general practice.

Another response of the doctor to the unconscious, regressively motivated search of the patient for a powerful, idolized, substitutive parent is to accept the assigned role. This may be reinforced by the doctor's unconscious wish to supersede the parent. The medical profession, with its responsibility for the patient's well-being and with its permissive, persuasive, and prohibitive aspects, lends itself particularly well to such an attitude. One doctor may undisguisedly treat his patients as if they were children, whereas another may adopt the Victorian principle that children should be seen but not heard (or, more precisely, not listened to), or may refrain from telling them what they want to know and what they are entitled to know. In this connection Balint's term "apostolic function" is relevant, for by it he means that doctors try to enforce, with apostolic zeal, their views on correct sick-role behavior.

Not only may a doctor adopt a substitutive parent function, actively and passively, in relation to his patients, but he may also reflect, and transfer to his patients, his own past attitudes to members of his own family. Some physicians devote themselves self-sacrificingly to the care of old ladies because they have had qualms about the surgeon's advice to operate, or have feared that even a well-considered operation might result in death. The treatment of members of one's family is generally avoided on the grounds that one's objectivity is impaired if one is emotionally involved. Actually, apart from incestuous implications, a doctor who does not dare to treat a sick member of his family is afraid of the negative aspects of his ambivalent relationship to the person in question.

When the doctor's neurotic conflicts definitely interpose themselves in the professional relationship, treatment may reach a stalemate. Even if the doctor sees the conflict in his patient, he may not be able to take appropriate action because his own similar conflicts contaminate the relationship. As a result, the doctor, unaware of his motivations, may induce the patient to act in accordance with his own unconscious needs. One doctor maintained the apparent happiness of his own marriage by advocating divorce as a solution for a patient's marital conflicts. Also, a doctor's neurotic conflict may prematurely terminate the treatment. On such occasions, doctor and patient usually seem to be in collusion to go no further. Often, after the doctor describes the encouraging opening phases of treatment, the patient seems to fade away.

Conclusion

In this general outline of the emotional problems of the physically ill and of the doctors who treat them, some aspects of the doctor-patient relationship have been chosen for presentation because the doctor's handling of patients, irrespective of the nature of their diseases and of his own motivations, represents the core of the psychiatric role of the general practitioner. Deliberately I have abstained from dealing with such specific issues as psychotics, neurotics, psychosomatic patients, the aged, the mentally defective, or delinquents. These areas have been admirably covered by many eminent writers. Reference may be made to Maurice Levine's *Psychotherapy in Medical Practice* (6); Knight Aldrich's "Psychoneuroses and Their Management in General Practice" (1); Brian Bird's *Talking with Patients* (3); Michael Balint's *The Doctor, His Patient, and the Illness* (2); and "The Doctor-Patient Relationship with Its Historical Context," by Marc H. Hollender, W. F. Knopf, and T. S. Szasz (5).

THE PSYCHIATRIC ROLE OF THE GENERAL PRACTITIONER

Everybody agrees with the *nil nocere* principle, though it is more easily stated than adhered to. Maurice Levine (6) has drawn up a list of five common mistakes made by general practitioners: (1) unnecessary operations; (2) too-frequent use of drugs, which may lead to drug addiction; (3) threats to patients regarding their sexual activity and aggressive misbehavior; (4) the use of domination to overcome a patient's neurotic anxiety; and (5) the arousal of anxiety without specific purpose.

In my view the main psychiatric role of the general practitioner is to understand himself, his patient, and the patient-doctor interaction. The much-advocated common-sense approach to these problems is not good enough. The so-called art of medicine is understandable, analyzable, teachable, and learnable. The argument that understanding of interactional processes interferes with intuitive action is valid to some extent, but it is still true that a doctor who understands why he does what he does, can do a better job than a doctor who is guided solely by intuition and common sense.

Diagnosis should cover the presence and the nature of emotional maladjustment on conscious, preconscious, and unconscious levels. General practitioners still have a long way to go before they will be able to do this.

For the treatment of psychological disorders or of psychological components of organic diseases, the general practitioner must make an intelligent self-assessment of the limitations of his knowledge and skill. Nobody in his right mind would seriously suggest that a general practitioner perform an appendectomy without adequate training. Unless there are psychiatric emergencies, or except in remote rural areas, general practitioners should not treat major psychological disorders. Treatment of such cases should be entrusted only to specifically trained doctors, or should be handled only with the coöperation or under the supervision of those so trained.

The argument that the general practitioner, who sees mental disorders in early stages and is acquainted with the intrafamilial situation, can nip such disorders in the bud is almost certainly fallacious. The family physician of bygone days has become a rare specimen, and incipient mental disorders are not easily amenable to treatment. It is true, however, that the general practitioner frequently encounters transient, stress-conditioned neurotic phenomena with which he can adequately deal.

Psychopharmacotherapy is undoubtedly of considerable benefit, though no mental conflict has ever been solved by drugs. The ever-lengthening list of phrenotropic drugs is puzzling enough for the experienced psychiatrist, and it must be even more so for the general practitioner. Much harm can be done by the indiscriminate use of phrenotropic drugs, and the general practitioner would be well advised to prescribe them only after consultation with a psychiatrist.

What psychotherapeutic measures can and should be adopted by the general practitioner? There are a number of things he can do: (1) he may be of great help to his patients by listening to them; (2) he may, by giving explanations and reassurances on the basis of his scientific knowledge, often allay unwarranted fears or, if he has tolerance and understanding, even morbid anxieties; (3) he can separate rational and irrational worries; (4) he can sort out the social difficulties of a patient, though caution must be used in giving advice and guidance, or in planning environmental manipulation, because the patient's difficulties may be the effect rather than the cause of the emotional disorder; (5) he may, by giving explanatory talks to members of the family, greatly alleviate the patient's lot; and (6) he can refer patients who are beyond his skill and knowledge to a psychiatrist.

PRACTICAL SUGGESTIONS

Training at medical schools. There is no doubt that medical schools leave much to be desired in training their students to deal with the human factor in disease. It remains to be seen to what extent the great increase in time given to the teaching of psychiatry in medical schools will affect the practitioner's role in the patient-doctor relationship. It is one thing to impart factual knowledge about, and intellectual understanding of, this relationship; it is quite another to teach a would-be doctor an awareness of himself and the capacity to empathize. Balint has suggested that certain students might be selected to participate in ongoing clinical seminars throughout their medical training. This approach, however, would have its limitations, for medical students and residents in hospitals rarely see patients in an ongoing relationship. It is only when a doctor takes up his own practice that the study of his patients' emotional conflicts and of his relationship to his patients receives an impetus. Then the doctor must devise his own solutions, or acquire more formal instruction.

Ongoing seminars for doctors in practice. The ongoing seminar originated with Balint at the Tavistock Clinic in England, and is now used in several centers in the United States and Canada, as well as in other countries. Pittenger reports on such a course as conducted in Pittsburgh for the past six years (10). Groups of about ten doctors each meet with a psychiatrist once a week and discuss their patients. The aim is to understand the nature of the patients' emotional conflicts and of the doctor-patient relationship, and the manner in which the doctor can use himself in his treatment. Self-awareness and the capacity to empathize are stressed in these seminars. Doctors attend for a period of months, or even of years. Because of the time between sessions, and the over-all duration of the course, they can test out new insights gained in the seminars. They also have the opportunity to work through many problems that arise in the psychological field.

Refresher courses. Refresher courses for general practitioners convey factual information and, moreover, give doctors confidence in handling their emotionally disturbed patients. A refresher course lasting a few days, however, cannot be expected to produce a fundamental change in a doctor's capacity to understand his patients or his interaction with them; it may even be detrimental by increasing a doctor's tendency to adopt an intellectualized approach to his patients. The doctor may be reassured if he can make an accurate descriptive diagnosis, but the diagnostic label does not necessarily help in handling a patient.

The psychiatrist as a consultant. Within the framework of the psychiatrist's relationship with the general practitioner, certain shifts in emphasis might well improve the handling of emotionally disturbed patients. If a number of general practitioners work in close association with a psychiatrist, and have ample opportunity to consult with one another, they may be able to achieve a more appropriate division of labor in keeping with their skills and treatment resources. There are three possible categories of patient management implicit in this plan:

1. Patients may be referred to the psychiatrist for total treatment.

2. Patients may be referred to the psychiatrist for consultation. Some of them may end up by taking total treatment from the psychiatrist. Others may continue with their regular practitioners, who will be helped in clarifying the diagnosis, the psychodynamics, or the main area of treatment by the patient's consultation with the psychiatrist. The general practitioner will be better able to formulate his treatment plan, and further consultations between him and the psychiatrist may be in the nature of supervisory sessions.

3. Patients may be returned to the care of the general practitioner after the psychiatrist has completed a phase of the treatment which requires his skill or his facilities. By freeing himself from spending time in following some patients throughout the treatment, the psychiatrist may find time to supervise the general practitioners.

These readjustments in the psychiatric role may enable the general practitioner to narrow the gap between himself and the psychiatrist, to the benefit of a larger number of patients.

REFERENCES

1. ALDRICH, G. KNIGHT. Psychoneuroses and their management in general practice. J. Chronic Dis., 9:212–219, 1959.
2. BALINT, MICHAEL. The doctor, his patient, and the illness. New York, International Universities Press, 1957.
3. BIRD, BRIAN. Talking with patients. Montreal, J. F. Lippincott, 1955.
4. FERENCZI, SANDOR. Disease—or patho-neuroses, *in* The theory and technique of psycho-analysis. London, The Hogarth Press and the Institute of Psycho-Analysis, 1950.
5. HOLLENDER, MARC H., W. F. KNOPF, and T. S. SZASZ. The doctor-patient relationship and its historical context. Am. J. Psychiat., 115:522, 1958.
6. LEVINE, MAURICE. Psychotherapy in medical practice. New York, Macmillan, 1952.
7. MARCONDES, DURVAL. New aspects of the clinical interview: countertransference difficulties. Psychosom. Med., XXII:211, 1960.
8. MENNINGER, KARL. Psychological factors in the choice of medicine as a profession. Bull. Menninger Clinic, 21 (no. 2):51, 1957.
9. NUNBERG, H. Practice and theory of psychoanalysis. Nervous and mental disease monographs, no. 74. New York, 1948.
10. PITTENGER, REX A. A method of training physicians in psychotherapy. Delivered at APA meeting, May, 1960.

11. REISER, M. F. Emotional aspects of cardiac disease. Am. J. Psychiat., 107:781, 1950–1951.
12. SIMMEL, E. The doctor-game, illness and the profession of medicine. Intern. J. Psychoanal., 7, 1926.
13. STAINBROOK, E. The community of the psychiatric patient, *in* American handbook of psychiatry, ed. S. Arieti. New York, Basic Books, 1959. Vol. I, chap. 6.

10 PERSONALITY DEVELOPMENT AND CHILDHOOD BEHAVIORAL DISABILITIES

BY GEORGE E. GARDNER, PH.D., M.D.

IN APPROACHING THIS SUBJECT I had three alternatives: first, to make a straight, factual presentation of a clinical case on the basis of which concepts could later be outlined in respect to the relationship of child development to the psychopathology in that case, with perhaps fruitful generalizations applicable to other behavioral disabilities of childhood; second, to summarize principles underlying the present-day child psychiatrist's clinical approach and his use of a developmental frame of reference, which could be delineated in tentative outline form; or, third, to use an effective combination of the "developmental age" approach and short illustrative case excerpts to highlight a number of immaturation points or faults in personality structure.

I chose to set aside the single-case and the case-excerpt methods, and to summarize tentatively, but as concisely as possible, the principles of the genetic approach and the critical developmental tasks and crises that children normally face. This brings us to the dissection and exposure of our clinical approach, for our own clarification and for the positing of future research needs for added content and added precision in age localization.

My perennial interest in this problem of relating development to specific clinical syndromes extends back thirty-one years, to the time when I had only the psychoanalytic literature plus personal communication afforded me by Dr. Ives Hendrick. I then published a paper entitled "The Measurement of the Psychotic Age," because it seemed to me that it was sensible, logical, clinically useful, and possible to locate the immaturation or regression point of the various schizophrenic types and the manic-depressive expressions at the various phases, month by month, in infant libidinal development. The necessary psychoanalytic data were in the literature, and it seemed that only a systemization of them was needed. (Needless to say, I relied very heavily upon the work of Abraham and Bernfeld.) I think, too, that I had in mind the notion that a more carefully worked out "psychotic age" in the obviously clear cases, but particularly in the seemingly mixed or clinically nonclassical cases, would give a more accurate clue to the probable chronicity or recoverability of the patient. At any rate, I took on the task of chronological age localization, and did it to my own satisfaction (though to the obvious indifference of almost everyone else).

Some ten or twelve years later, after I had become

acquainted with the behavioral deviations in children, I stressed a necessary search for the developmental location and evaluation of the "pseudopsychotic nucleus" in such cases. I must then have had the same objective in mind: to ascertain the relationship of child development to later psychopathology. This, of course, has always been basic to the psychoanalytic approach to the understanding of human behavior.

In the past ten years my interest in this approach has increased. At the present moment I optimistically detect the possibility that temporal relationships between phases of development and specific primary or allied (secondary) disabling symptoms and syndromes in child behavior will be more and more accurately outlined. In the past decade we have been driving fast toward clinical application of this dyadic "development-disability" relationship. Many clinically oriented research programs in child development are now in progress in some of our very best child psychiatry units.

It is particularly significant to me that these developmental studies are no longer solely concerned with the elucidation of specific stages in development in infancy. Their range has been extended under the impact of ego psychology data, and they are now concerned also with the possibility of more accurate localization of specific discrete stages in ego development after infancy and the preschool years.

An added stimulus to my interest in the further clarification of the development-disability relationship is the almost hopeless chaos of the diagnostic classifications of a majority of the behavioral disabilities of childhood, and the lack of an accurate nomenclature. A number of national committees are concerned with this important problem, and many child psychiatry clinics, as well, are now addressing themselves to the task.

Perhaps the best possible system of nosology would be one that relates the primary and secondary childhood disabilities at any age level, as directly and as definitely as our increasing knowledge will allow, to an age-located personality development task failure. I refer to failures in varying tasks that present themselves seriatim to the child for solution at every age level through adolescence. This involves, of course, our continuing interest in the ego-confronted tasks of the latency period—a stage in development where age localization has not yet been seriously attempted. The complexities in diagnosis and prognosis seem to arise from the fact that every clinical syndrome is enmeshed, sometimes almost inextricably, in a matrix that demonstrates wide variations (a zigzag profile) in maturity or lack of maturity for the particular chronological age of the individual child patient.

Yet we must continue to tease out for high-power examination and age localization the multiple and multivariable, and sometimes certainly minute and subtle, nucleolar developmental task solutions that eventually comprise the basic energic structure complexes of the mind. We must study the id motivational drive segments, the highly distinctive and disparate units of the control-defense and executive ego, and its specialized unconscious unit, the superego (ego ideal). We shall then be well on our way to establishing useful temporal norms or narrowed age ranges for a system of diagnosis in terms of developmental age task failures. Obviously, we must at the same time continue in our discoveries, and precise location, of the developmental tasks presented to the child for solution throughout the whole range of ego development.

It is to a consideration of these problems that I now turn. I shall summarize the basic principles underlying the tasks set for the developing infant and child. We need more and more accurate age localization to give significance to the clinical material. There need not be unanimity of opinion concerning the principles I cite, nor concerning the elucidation of developmental tasks. What we are most interested in is emphasis (in reality a reëmphasis) on, and an extension of, the psychoanalytic approach used by our clinical specialty.

BASIC PRINCIPLES IN DEVELOPMENTAL AGE– DISABILITY STUDY

The premise most basic to all our work is that behavioral disabilities in childhood can be experientially induced or created through the anxiety-provoking threats, stresses, and crises that confront the child, as well as by the deleterious effects of an unfavorable interpersonal milieu characterized by the presence of nonempathetic and nonsympathetic (yet to the child highly significant) human beings.

No doubt inheritance, constitutional diatheses, or metabolic, glandular biochemical dysfunctions are the determinants of many atypical or abnormal conditions. There is room in our theoretical acceptance for genuinely serious consideration of these premises, and research along these lines will be intensive and exhaustive. Nonetheless, we who are child therapists and/or child analysts assume in our clinical work and in our research that children subjected to certain experiences will become behaviorally disabled and that, in turn, if they are subjected to other or favorably altered interpersonal experiences, the disabilities will be modified or eliminated. Some of our more specific assumptions may, perhaps, with rewording or rephrasing, or with differing emphases, be accepted by all of us.

As clinicians we may assume that there are three basic, innate drives in all organisms. The first is the drive to live, or the basic drive to avoid death, either complete death or partial death through mutilation of the body. The second basic drive inherent in all organic life is the drive to die; it is, of course, in opposition to the first. The inner drive to die may be expressed (1) by actual destruction of the body or body parts or by a contrived destruction through a selected agency in the environment; or (2) by the ever-present process of selecting lower and lower (or more primitive) organizations of behavioral responses and modes or patterns of living. This latter expression of the death drive subserves the mechanism of regression. The third drive is the libidinal or sexual drive. It is aimed at procreation of the species and is an integral part of, or inextricably allied with, the drive to live.

Anticipating my later discussion of certain developmental tasks in early infancy, we may make the assumption that these three drives (life, death, sex) are motivated and energized by phylogenetically built-in body processes. There is a gradual, seriatim, neurophysiological growth pattern in the emergence of these scores of media (particularly in the motoric pleasure sequences). At differing levels of infancy and childhood, the organism assigns different values, in a hierarchical ascendancy of importance, to certain of these body-process pleasures. These pleasures are not by any means confined solely to the ascendancies and sequences so familiar to us and so clinically valuable to us, which relate to the gastrointestinal and gastrourinary tracts. For example, we tend to overlook or undervalue the pleasure sequences that are inherent in the musculoarticulatory systems.

It is relatively easy to list the scores of body processes which are indeed pleasurable, but it is equally easy to overlook the important fact that every one of them also has the inherent power to elicit the feeling of pain. The pain results not only when the processes cannot be expressed—that is, when they are repressed—but also when they are expressed or activated in excessive degree. When potential excesses in expression are used in the service of the drive toward death or of sadomasochistic control impulses toward others, or in the interest of self-initiated punitive impulses, their clinical significance is by no means unimportant.

In the light of the well-established principles relative to a necessary adjustive, adaptive, and defensive continuum in respect to the cellular, the organic, and the interorganic functioning of the body, we may postulate similar homeostatic continuums at the higher developmental behavioral levels. These continuums relate both to pleasure-pain processes and to the symbolic life-death processes. All the principles of cellular pathology—including those that relate to defensive responses in acute or chronic inflammation, to physiological and structural regressions in psychosomatic conditions, and certainly to type-designated reactions based on a relative primitivism of cellular response used to differentiate benign and malignant cellular responses in neoplastic diseases—have pertinent counterparts in behavioral disorders, such as neuroses and psychoses. Parsimony in respect to nature's responses leads to the expectation that at any organizational level the organism's pathological responses, including the behavioral, are prototypical (paratypes one of the other), even though we are dealing at one level with cells and at another with behavior.

Two important theoretical points emphasize the compelling need to search for, and use, accurate age localization of a discrete behavioral symptom or of a behavioral disability syndrome, as well as accurate developmental placement of clear-cut neurotic states (phobias, obsessive compulsive states) on the age scale of psychosexual development. The first point is that each symptom—isolated and single, or in combination with associated symptoms—has its own specific age localization as a developmental fault. Second, we may assume, borrowing from cellular pathology, that the lower in the age scale of personality development the single symptom-fault or syndrome-fault was inculcated, the more seriously meaningful it is for present adjustment and also for the solution of developmental tasks at future age levels. In short, if these borrowed concepts are indeed applicable in our field, we can establish a clinically oriented body of knowledge which in essence will be a science of childhood behavioral pathology.

Another basic principle is that all the behavioral and emotional deviations or disabilities in childhood constitute the best possible, and perhaps the only, effective compromise responses, or compromise life pattern or life plan, in the presence of severe internalized or external conflicts, which the child organism can make to ensure life and to avoid death. It is clinically useful, therefore, in our interpretations of affect responses in earliest infancy (which are capable of being reactivated forever after), to assume that the feeling of pleasure is the basic nonverbal equivalent in the baby or the preschool child of the concept of life and living, of being alive. Upon this all later verbal concepts of life and being alive are built. Conversely, the feeling of pain, or of the lack of pleasure, in the infant is the basic nonverbal equivalent of the feeling of impending death and destruction. Upon this feeling and its ingredients is based and built the mature concept of death as inevitable. Possibly more accurately, the young child's concept of impending or possible death is owing to his actual or fantasied abandonment by biologically significant humans in his life (loss of a love object). It is probably built upon the displeasure feeling of body process, whereas the concept of possible or impending mutilation is based upon the feeling of pain. No doubt the preverbal mental (central nervous system) representation of life and living includes an awareness of the pleasurable expression of certain body processes, and the preverbal mental representation of death and dying is somehow related either to the blocked expression of pleasurable body processes or to the painful excess of expression of the same body processes.

The child's crucially important feeling of anxiety, his panic reaction, is an awareness of the helplessness and the feeling of vulnerability which follow the realization that the expression of desired body pleasures has been blocked, or the realization that the excess point of pleasurable expression is now approaching pain. Anxiety as a signal for the mobilization and utilization of effective defenses is the definitive correlate of the signal meaning of pain at the cellular level. This in turn calls forth the body's multiple defensive maneuvers to maintain life and tissue integrity.

The child senses that possible impending death or mutilation, signaled by anxiety caused by the feelings of helplessness and vulnerability, may be mediated by (1) a significant person or an animal, material object, or "nature" symbol of that significant person for the expression of forbidden body-process pleasures; (2) another significant person in recompense for the child's own mutilative or death wishes toward this human love object; or (3) destruction or mutilation at one's own hand, such as self-punishing devices, accident milieu settings, and the carrying out of games and self-contrived "sports" of daring where the brink of death may be close.

Clinical evidence has taught us that all the love-object relationships of the child to other humans and, indeed, to the child's self-image as regards his body and its parts, are inevitably placed on a sadomasochistic continuum. The necessary frustrations exercised by others, even in the interest of the child's physical safety, or by the child himself, make for this inevitability. There is never complete unmodified love or complete unmodified hatred even in a child's most crucial love-object relationships. Two important questions are posed in quantifying and qualitating this factor: (1) To what degree is this dyadic relationship disabling? (2) What are its basic meanings referable to control (from guidance to dependent seduction or slavery) or to death (abandonment, rejection, mutilation)?

The child from infancy onward continues to establish within himself a hierarcy or a gradient of ascribed values in reference to the significance of the people who populate his life at any particular chronological stage. The relative position in importance of "significant people" varies as the child develops. At first, of course, the humans of greatest significance are those who have biological significance: primarily the mother, secondarily the father and the siblings, and later other relatives and close friends of the family. Later on, if the child's development is orderly, individual peer-group members, teachers, and leaders in play, in camp, in supervised recreation, or in church and community activities assume prominence in the significance hierarchy. This echeloning of persons on value levels of significance continues throughout childhood and, indeed, adolescent and adult life.

From earliest infancy through adolescence, each change in response demanded in the furtherance of behavioral growth, personality development, and learning arouses at least a minimum of anxiety feeling. This is particularly true in respect to changes that may threaten, or seem to threaten, the stability and the security value of the child's love-object relationships. Such anxiety may be fleeting or nondisabling, phasically disabling for a relatively short period, or significantly and lastingly disabling to the point where a protective regression to a lower stage of behavioral organization may result in the interest of reduction of anxiety and reëstablishment of a feeling of security.

A related but yet distinct clinical postulate is the assumption that all growth, all development (embryonic and cellular as well as behavioral), and all learning depend on the ability of the organism at all these differing levels of response to make the effective and efficient differentiation of responses. All behavioral responses, if they are set in motion by the demand for change and growth, must proceed from the more undifferentiated to the more particularized. Contrast the potentiated screaming and screeching of Maria Callas as an infant with her exquisitely differentiated vocal performance of an aria at the Metropolitan Opera House thirty years later. But such differentiation, however subtle, is always accompanied by a modicum of anxiety which is potentially disabling.

As a modification of my claim that only differentiation ensures growth, consider the possibly overriding demand that the ego must be able (without disabling anxiety) to appraise a newly presented problem requiring change and differentiation. The child must weigh the problem realistically as a stimulus that may require a sameness of response rather than differentiation. Studies dealing with embryonic and paranatal development, however, indicate that a progressive differentiation and refinement of response is necessary in all growth. It is an important function of the child's ego, in reference to all demanded responses, to be free enough from anxiety to maintain flexibility in comparative evaluations of stimuli. It must, in each instance, determine what elements the situation at the moment has in common with previous situations that demanded responses, and whether a similar response, under the conditioned-response formula, or an essentially new differentiated response is called for. This maintenance of flexibility in evaluation and action is one of the criteria that we may apply in estimating the child's ego strength.

Inasmuch as we are concerned at this point with problems that relate to the learning process, and, specifically, with a continuum position of anxiety in the face of every demand for change, let us recall the observations of the behavioristic school of the 1920's. The behaviorists said that the feeling underlying curiosity stemmed from a conflict, momentary or prolonged, among possible responses, and that the feeling tone designated as curiosity had within it many elements in common with the feeling tone characteristic of anxiety. This notion, if correct, could have considerable meaning for clinical research personnel who deal with severe emotionally determined educational achievement blocks.

Most of us subscribe to the clinically demonstrable fact that the ability of children to cope with potentially anxietygenic traumata or milieu varies greatly, even in siblings when exposed to essentially the same traumata or to a similarly deleterious environment. The variation in effectiveness may be observed in any one child as he faces different tasks presented to him at different chronological ages. We are often amazed at the frustration tolerance and at the acuteness or lack of acuteness, in the sense of vulnerability, which different children demonstrate in seemingly identical situations. The child who always "escapes" intrigues us, even though we can find sensible psychodynamic explanations for one child's failure to cope when his siblings serenely, even triumphantly, solve similar tasks in personality development. In such instances we can, to our own satisfaction, posit subtle differences in milieu—differences created by the differing ordinal position of the patient, or differences in the attitudes and child-rearing practices of the mother. Yet no one has so far deliberately undertaken a well-designed, clinically intensive study of these escapees.

The clinical assumptions I have outlined are derived from, and in turn are applicable to, the adequate solution or the mis-, mal-, or nonsolution of a series of tasks in personality development posited for the child at various chronological age levels. Included also in the concept of such tasks are allied concepts of stages or phases in development, and resultant realizations and evaluations by the child in respect to himself and to the human and nonhuman world that sets the tasks for him, plus an observation of the consequences of his successes or his failures.

One of the various parameters of personality development concerns itself with the development of effective or defective interpersonal relationships, the crucial relatedness or nonrelatedness of the child to other persons. While listing some of the tasks set within this parameter, we recall that failure in any task solution at each age level may be related to a diagnosable major or minor disability of a phasic or permanent nature. The list does not aim at completeness or at accurate temporal pinpointing of tasks in respect to localization. Expansion of the list and further localization will be attempted as we amass a larger and larger body of knowledge in normal child development and in child-behavior pathology. In the face of accepted overlapping in time, we can merely arrange the tasks in tentative chronological order in respect to (1) infancy and the preschool period, (2) the "mastery" or latency period, and (3) adolescence.

TASKS AND STAGES IN PERSONALITY DEVELOPMENT

In order to account for even the most primitive ego formations in the child, we assume that he has paranatally (1) an intact, though by no means completely developed, sensorimotor system; and (2) a large number of the subsequent functioning or potentially functioning body processes that simultaneously sustain life and afford the attendant feelings of pleasure which motivate repetitive expression. We also assume a postnatal period in which disparate and diffuse id responses are given without the infant's being able to differentiate between his body and the objects about him. In this stage of "fusion," presumably, objects seem to be adherent extensions of the infant's body.

PLEASURABLE BODY PROCESSES, STATES, AND ACTIONS

I. *Visual*
1. Looking
2. Seeing
3. Blinking
4. Rolling eyes

II. *Auditory*
5. Hearing
    a) Self
    b) Others

III. *Olfactory*
6. Smelling
7. Sniffing

IV. *Oral*
8. Tasting
9. Sucking
10. Mouthing
11. Tonguing
12. Lipping

IV. *Oral (continued)*
  13. Lapping
  14. Retaining
  15. Spitting
  16. Drooling
  17. Belching
  18. Biting
  19. Grinding teeth
  20. Clenching teeth
  21. Clicking
    a) Tongue
    b) Teeth
  22. Bubbling
V. *Vocalizing*
  23. Babbling
  24. Humming
  25. Groaning
  26. Screaming
  27. Laughing
  28. Crying
  29. Talking
VI. *Respiratory*
  30. Inspiration
  31. Expiration
  32. Blowing
  33. Coughing
  34. Sneezing
  35. Choking
  36. Holding breath
  37. Sighing
  38. Yawning
  39. Eructation
VII. *Of the gastrointestinal tract*
  40. Swallowing

41. ⎰ Vomiting ⎱ Ejecting
42. Retention
43. ⎰ Excreting ⎱ Emptying
44. Expelling
VIII. *Of the genitourinary tract*
  45. Retention
  46. Urinating
  47. Erecting
  48. Incorporating
IX. *Related to skin, mucous membrane, and hair*
  49. Covering
  50. Exposing
  51. Wrinkling
  52. Contacting
  53. Rubbing
  54. Scratching
  55. Stroking
  56. Smearing
X. *Motor*
  57. Grasping
  58. Clenching
  59. Crushing
  60. Poking
  61. Pinching
  62. Pushing
  63. Pulling
  64. Patting
  65. Hooking
  66. Inserting
  67. Holding
  68. Hitting
  69. Punching

x. *Motor* (*continued*)
70. Slapping
71. Clinging
72. Throwing
73. Pounding
74. Elbowing
75. Shouldering
76. Lifting
77. Dropping
78. Carrying
79. Swaying
80. Bending
81. Rolling
82. Crawling
83. Creeping
84. Sitting
85. Standing
86. Falling
87. Bouncing
88. Banging
89. Jumping
90. Walking
91. Running
92. Tiptoeing
93. Stamping
94. Kneeling
95. Kneeing
96. Sliding
97. Kicking
98. Smiling
99. Frowning
100. Grimacing
101. Vestibular changes (loss and recovery of balance)
102. Sleeping
103. Rocking
104. Climbing

It is useful to consider the ego in its development as comprising a series of time-placed, solved task segments. My purpose now is to reëmphasize the possibilities in a developmental age approach by a componental analysis, hoping that other research workers may reorder, expand, and age-localize the components.

THE ESTABLISHMENT OF A BODY-PROCESS-PLEASURE EGO

The body image. The establishment of a "complex" in the mind through closely associated pleasurable body sensations, with the simultaneous occurrence of varied sensations and the growing awareness of their relatedness, plus a positioning of them, gives rise to an "image" of definitely circumscribed sources of pleasure and pain.

The establishment of body boundaries. Coincidental with this evolving group of associated body-process sensations, there evolves the realization of the existence of substances or objects beyond and nonadherent to the surfaces and limits of the body. These experiences become the basic determinants of body boundaries, and they persistently combat the initial nondifferentiated fusion of the body with nonbody objects.

Self-initiation of body processes. With the establishment of the body image and an appreciation of body boundaries, there develops the all-important realization that pleasurable body processes can be self-initiated. That is, they can be set in operation by certain activities under the child's own control. From this moment on, the self-initiation of scores of pleasures is resorted to repeatedly, and almost compulsively.

Hierarchical preference positioning. Nearly seventy years of unchallengeable psychoanalytic data show that the child establishes a hierarchical preference positioning of certain groups of body areas and body processes, and that the pleasures associated with these groups are self-sought above all others. They become hypercathected, if you will, as the primary sources of autoerotic pleasures. The evidence points, of course, to the gradual, almost exclusive ascendancy in the galaxy of the possible self-initiated body-process pleasures afforded by the buccal cavity, the gastrointestinal system, and the genitourinary system. All the tasks and stages in personality development in the infant and preschool years are inextricably linked to, and are dependent upon, the time location of various stages in psychosexual development, such as oral, anal, phallic, and genital. They are of nuclear and primary importance. It is well to remember, however, that the other less frequently highlighted body systems, particularly the skin and the motoric system, with its host of potentially pleasurable responses, should not be relegated to relative unimportance in the child's mind.

Pleasures of the gastrointestinal and gastrourinary systems. The child very early realizes that, specifically, the dyad fullness-emptiness constitutes a continuum associated at either end with either pleasure or pain. The pleasure and the pain, in regard to the fullness or the emptiness of the hollow viscera, are, in turn, associated with pleasure and pain in respect to tension or release of tension. These biological bases of later-associated symbolic interpersonal-response transactions are extremely important clinically.

The sensation of pain. The child gradually realizes that all the body processes and states giving pleasure have inherent in them the power to create the sensation of pain because of (1) the absence of the possibility for expression, or (2) expression in excess.

Self-initiation of pleasure and pain. Because the child now realizes that he himself has the power to initiate both pleasure and pain through acts of stimulation, the bases are laid for the emergence of further critical realizations, concepts, attitudes, and feelings. (1) The success of the repetitiously self-sought and self-initiated body-process pleasures produces a state of primary narcissism and omnipotence. (2) On the other hand, the infant realizes that these processes can give pain as well as pleasure, and that he has the power to elicit either sensation. As a result, the basic concept of primary ambivalence emerges. (3) These two realizations taken together allow for a gradual and very important objectification of the body or of a body part, to the end that the body itself takes on the qualities of an external object. That the infant's body and its parts come to be regarded as an object, with ambivalent feelings of love and hate, is of no small consequence in respect to later clinical conditions. It is by no means unimportant at the time when the child takes the next step in ego development, that is, the establishment of relationships with other human objects, who have bodies not unlike his own.

THE EARLIEST LOVE-OBJECT-RELATED EGO

A second area of the infant's ego development involves the critical task of relating to other human beings. Certain related stages or steps seem necessary, and the failure to take them may result in maturation arrest or inculcated faults in the personality structure.

    1. The child soon realizes that both material and human objects can initiate or potentiate pleasures, or can be

used by him to initiate or potentiate pleasures. These are sought and used if they are adjacent to the child.

2. Soon, however, the child realizes that there is a definite hierarchy in the power of these different external objects to initiate pleasure, and that human objects have a marked ascendancy in value. In light of the quantity, the variety, the intensity, and the frequency of the pleasures elicited by and through human objects, nonhuman material objects, though still eagerly sought and repeatedly used, become secondary in importance. If the human object responds with need gratifications, the task of accomplishing a primary meaningful and lasting relatedness to a human love object has been successfully solved.

3. In the first months of relatedness to one human being, the mother, the child sets up (and later modifies) what could be termed a normal symbiotic relationship demanding body closeness and clinging, with the supervention of varying degrees of anxiety or panic when the one significant human being is absent or nonavailable. In this one person, and from her, there is the initial establishment of the all-important sense of security with, and basic trust in, love objects.

4. Here again, however, as in the infant's self-initiation of pleasure from his own body, he discovers that this "other initiator," the mother, does not always gratify needs and, indeed, that her acts and her absence can cause pain. The secondary ambivalence in respect to human love objects is necessarily inculcated in the child. The importance of this feeling is its relative effect upon, and its modification of, the child's basic trust.

5. The sense of trust and security in one significant person as a task accomplishment must next be extended and expanded to include other near and significant love objects in the family—father, siblings, relatives—and others in close relationships with them. This demands a drastic modification of the symbiotic or parasitic relationship to the mother, and of the disabling, paniclike reactions to her absence. In the first instance this modification causes a depressive response or longing for the temporarily lost love object. It also requires the ability on the part of the child to conjure up an image, or a hallucination, of the probable presence of the object or of its inevitable early return.

THE CONTROL SEGMENT OF THE EARLY EGO

Only in the milieu of security and trust in love objects is it possible for the child to establish the rudimentary but effective control and modification of the demand for immediate and complete gratification and for the unaltered expression of body-process pleasures. The task of accepting delay and frustration of these pleasures can be solved only at the point where the need for and the value of the continued love of the love object become greater than the value now placed upon self-initiated pleasures without regard to the mother's demands or displeasure. The development of the control segment of the ego, and of the basic rudiments of its specialized unconscious portion of this segment, the superego (ego ideal), presumably requires incorporated pictures of the person who demands control, and an identification of the self with and an expression of her aggressive acts, threatening facial expressions, and later her words of both admonition and praise.

After the establishment of these segments of the ego—the body-process ego or body image, the earliest love-object-related ego, and the control segments of the ego—they must be effectively unified into a sense of self with an accompanying sense of self-worth. The sense of self-worth is a very important double image in that it comprises the child's own image of his worth and an associated image of his worth and value in the eyes of the significant love objects near him. These "self" and "other" images are thereafter the child's constant preoccupation, and determine his ability to cope with the inevitable frustrations, threats, and stresses encountered throughout childhood. His diffuse and profuse identities are assumed in respect to these value images, and the momentary levels (the rise and fall) of his sense of security are measured in relation to their positive and negative aspects.

The Oedipus Complex

The all-consuming tasks in personality development in the periods of postinfancy (24–30 months) and prelatency (36 months to 5½ years) relate to the meaningful establishment of the Oedipal relationship with the parent of the opposite sex, and its successful resolution. There are many antecedents to the establishment of this relationship, and its course may be stormy or placid. Through this postinfancy expression of the insistent, compelling drive for total possession of the love of the parent of the opposite sex, the child, though he loses the main goal, emerges with basic part solutions to some very important tasks in personality development. Among these are (1) a relatively firm beginning realization of the existence of sex preferences and sex differences; (2) the initial clarification of the heterosexual aim and object orientation of the child's biologic equipment; (3) the initial, but usually thereafter firm, identification with his or her own sex and with the numerous roles that accompany it; and (4) an essential minimal bisexuality that gives the desired combination of masculine aggressiveness and feminine tenderness. These are by no means small or unimportant initial steps in the solution of continuing critical tasks. The establishment and resolution of the Oedipal situation is immensely important in preparing the child for effective solution of the tasks set for him in the latency period (5½ to 10½ or 11 years).

THE DEVELOPMENT TASKS IN THE LATENCY PERIOD

Psychoanalysts have provided adequate data in reference to the seriatim appearance of the important and critical tasks in development during the infancy and preschool periods. To construct our developmental scales and age localizations, we now need continued and intensive research for more and more exact age localization. In Boston alone, research being carried out by Mrs. Beata Rank, Dr. Samuel Kaplan, Dr. Eleanor Pavenstedt, Dr. Haskell Cohen, Dr. Geraldine Rickard, Dr. Peter Wolff, and Dr. Abraham Fineman, to name but a few, encourage optimism. Adjacent and related studies have been undertaken by Dr. Eric Lenneberg in speech, and by Drs. Felix Deutsch and Tully Benaron in cross-cultural pictographic material here and in Israel. Other valuable work is progressing in other child-analytic and child-psychiatry research centers. Most of these studies are being conducted by expert clinicians who take great pains to relate their findings to clinical states.

Let us consider the various task problems presented, their levels of appearance, their height, their modification in expression, and their final expression and solution in the latency period and adolescence. The difficulties attendant upon even a seriatim outline, owing to the individual complexities of the tasks, their overlapping in time, and their interrelationships with associated tasks, now become apparent. In respect to the profiled latency-period task failures, we are forced, again and again, to content ourselves with the diagnostic label, "primary behavior disorder."

We can, however, make a start toward a seriatim, if not a specific, age-level localization. The main tasks of the latency period are:

1. Continuing—and final—resolution of the Oedipus complex.

2. Modification of residual disabilities relating to penis envy in girls.

3. Modification of residual disabilities relating to the castration complex in boys.

4. Control of (*a*) destructive impulses and (*b*) seductive dependent impulses on the sadomasochistic dyad carried through from early infantile responses, plus the eradication of

death wishes directed at the parents because of need frustrations.

5. Impersonalization of the aggressive drives and the substitution of their modified, attenuated expression in (*a*) accepted rules of play, and (*b*) educational achievement.

6. The ability, without anxiety, to enter into satisfactory and satisfying relationships with peer-group members: (*a*) individuals, (*b*) small groups in clubs and in the classroom, and (*c*) large groups or crowds (the "market place").

7. Effective utilization of fantasy as a defense in the service of anxiety reduction.

8. Reduction of the anxiety-reducing fantasy so that it will not interfere with learning.

9. The substitution of an achievement fantasy for the anxiety-reducing fantasy. The achievement fantasy necessarily demands the acceptance of the crucial items exhibited by a future-oriented individual, as required in Western culture, and a drastic modification of present-day orientation. It may be true that almost all successful school learning is motivated by achievement fantasies.

10. Self-freeing, or being freed by others, from anxiety to the degree that habits conducive to precision learning can be inculcated.

11. The strengthening and consolidation, and particularly the impersonalization, of the superego (ego ideal).

12. Development of a property sense, accompanied by dissolution of the earlier concepts (*a*) that property is adherent to the body of the person, and hence is an object to be utilized for the expression of aggressive drives, or an object stolen as a symbol of the love of, or as a gift from, a significant love object, and (*b*) that property symbolizes body parts; and

by disassociation of the act of stealing (a) as a substitute for libidinal drives, and (b) as provocation for needed punishment for other forbidden acts. (At what age do we expect these impulses with their unconscious meaning to be at their height, at what age do we expect them to disappear, and what is their sequential order?)

13. Dissociation of repeated gifts as the sole or magnified interpersonal expression of love and acceptance, and of the lack of gifts as the indicator of rejection and loss of love.

14. Inculcation of the ability to share objects with others without a command or a demand by significant adults.

15. Strengthening of the already partly established identification with the roles of the child's own sex in respect to responses, interests, and orientation in a cross-sectional sense, and also with future sex roles. Here there are definite stages of growth: (a) phasic assumption of protective (anxiety-reducing) bisexuality in play and sometimes in work-at-home roles, and (b) use of reaction formation in mid-latency by both sexes to disclaim any meaningful identity with members of the opposite sex. (At what age before adolescence, and by what means, are these protective positions, feelings, and overt acts modified?)

16. Effective dissociation in the mind of the child of sadism (physical assault) and sexual love.

17. Modification of the child's unconscious self-image as a possible destructive, mutilative, or sickness-endowing agent in respect to either parent. This task is closely associated with the task of overcoming the unconscious fear that injury or death will befall a parent if the child does wrong.

18. Modification of the child's interpersonal value systems, which have categorized people as either (a) totally

bad, sinful, and threatening, or (*b*) totally good, righteous, and loving. (At what age does the child place persons in only one of these categories? Do fairy stories, comic books, television, and radio affect the recognition that persons are both good and bad?)

19. Modification of both the symbolic-protective and the aggressive use of and belief in the power of magical and ritualistic words, thoughts, actions, and mannerisms. A continuation of such beliefs, because of heightened anxiety levels, creates learning blocks or leads to underachievement.

20. Relinquishment by the girl of the primitive belief that (*a*) pregnancy can be initiated by the oral route, (*b*) gestation takes in a portion of the gastrointestinal tract, and (*c*) babies are born via the anal canal. This necessitates a rudimentary (but corrective) differentiation of the gastrointestinal and genitourinary tracts.

21. Acquisition by the boy of similar corrective medical information, together with acceptance of the fact that he cannot some day become a female or give birth to babies.

22. Acceptance of the designated authority positions of significant figures beyond the home: adults or peer-group members.

23. Elimination of separation anxiety in respect to absence or loss of either family or nonfamily group members.

The child faces these developmental personality tasks in the period of mastery of his impulses and of his human and nonhuman world. The duty of child psychiatrists and child analysts is to add to this list of tasks from clinical experience, and to determine accurate age levels for their emergence and solution.

TASKS OF PERSONALITY
DEVELOPMENT
IN ADOLESCENCE

I shall not go into extensive detail here in regard to the analysis of component parts of the developmental tasks presented to children at puberty and adolescence. I have already published some of my observations on this subject (1). I shall, however, describe the general tasks that are deemed important. Five major tasks confront the child as he enters his adolescent years, and numerous tasks of a subsidiary nature may be subsumed under the five.

1. Modification of unconscious concepts of parental figures. This extremely difficult task must be solved if subsequent steps in development are to be achieved. This is not solely a "drive for independence," as it is sometimes called, but an extensive alteration of the frames of guidance in behavior which have been strong structural elements in the child's personality. The young child's security is predicated upon the all-knowingness and the all-powerfulness of his mother and father, which have been accepted as his own strength, as a reliable guide, and as protection against his own impulses and the actions of others.

But reliance on the alleged omniscience and omnipotence of the parents cannot be maintained. Through his many experiences within and outside the home, the child repeatedly sees evidence to the contrary, and he is beset by the anxiety of insecurity. This is just as well, for otherwise his faith in the omniscience and the omnipotence of his parents might act as an immovable counterstimulus to growth and development. Nonetheless, it is difficult for the adolescent to modify these concepts, or, rather, it is difficult for him to find substitutes for his parents in this regard. He tries desperately, as many a harassed parent of an adolescent can attest, to place another person (indeed, almost any other person) in the parent's role as the supreme counselor. But the effort is doomed to failure, because nobody is omniscient and nobody is omnipotent. Moreover, in the last analysis, whatever knowingness or power adolescents achieve in the process of becoming adult must be impersonalized and must reside within themselves as a part of their self-concept, as self-directed and not other-directed.

A sometimes disastrous devaluation of parents may take place during this necessary stage of development. Adolescents, and indeed adults who are still essentially adolescent, are extremely vulnerable to the seductive voice of the false leader, or of the leader with false ideology or intent. Adolescents (of whatever chronological age) respond to such a leader because he poses as an omniscient person who can do their thinking for them, and as an omnipotent person who will be their power.

This formidable task of deauthoritizing and impersonalizing the controls over one's behavior may never be achieved, and if achieved it must thereafter be repeatedly reachieved. In any event, the first and crucial step toward achievement must be taken in adolescence.

2. Identification with sex role. The second task, which may generate serious conflicts, is the child's identification with the sex role for which he or she was biologically determined. The pressures that impinge upon the child, from the parental society to the political society, demand completion of this task. This identification is not limited merely to the biological sex role to be assumed in adult life, but includes also all the roles, dominant and subsidiary, which society insists upon. In view of the dangers, actual or alleged, factual or fanciful, which confront youth, and the ignorance in respect to sex roles, it is surprising that adolescents ever perform this developmental task and become reasonably conflict-free adults. That they do grow up and assume the proper sex roles is owing more to their innate resilience, their dissatisfaction with half-truths or nontruths, and to their curiosity, than it is to the guidance they receive from adults.

3. Modification of fear of heterosexual love relationships. This task is allied to the first two tasks I have named. There must be a modification of the reactivated earlier unconscious dread that a lasting heterosexual love relationship means total subjugation for oneself. This dread is a reactivation of the unconscious infancy fears of (or wishes for) omnipotent and omniscient control by the parents, and of the unconscious fear or wish that a lasting heterosexual relationship may result in the assumption by oneself of omnipotent control over the love object. In consequence of their inevitable reactivation in adolescence, these early tasks of childhood and their attendant conflicts have to be faced anew and finally solved realistically, through modification. Occasionally, successful resolutions of unconscious conflicts, relative to dread of an inevitable enslavement of oneself by the love object or of the inevitable enslavement of the love object by oneself, are not made in adolescence. This is the reason that many analysts have to deal with interpersonal maladjustments characterized by neurotically driven, repetitive, unconsciously contrived love-object losses and dismissals.

4. *Assumption of standards of morality.* A specific segment of the last-named over-all task is the assumption of standards of morality which are acceptable and appropriate to contemporary adult society. From society's point of view the needs are obvious. I want to emphasize the adolescent's need for inner controls, not only in regard to sexual behavior, but in all the roles the individual must play in his associations in society. The adolescent wants and needs universally agreed-upon and universally adhered-to fixed and unchallengeable standards of social conduct. Even more does he need agreed-upon standards that do not repeatedly disrupt his personality through the insecurities attendant upon impossibility of attainment. To imply that the adolescent is faced with difficult tasks and with serious conflicts in regard to both tenets and models, as he tries to discern and assimilate such standards, is a gross understatement.

5. *Decisions as to education and vocation.* In the choice of education and vocation, adolescents frequently have serious inner conflicts. The conscious choices ultimately ar-

rived at are probably determined, again with attendant serious conflicts, by deep unconscious needs. These in themselves would be conflictive enough. But the conflict is compounded by the multitudinous pressures and the varying value ratings, in respect to occupations, which arise from ethnic, family, school, community, and peer groups. Adolescents believe that some of the choices made are irreversible, and that in making them they have committed themselves to follow certain circumscribed courses, forever forsaking others. If it is true, as alleged by Freud, that adult adjustment and maturity are determined in large part by the ability to love and the ability to work, the successful solution of educational and vocational problems is a major accomplishment for an adolescent, comparable only to the assumption of the role consistent with his or her sex.

In the face of these five serious tasks, and of others that might be cited, what is the characteristic response we expect from adolescents, and, indeed, almost always find? Adolescence is a temporary stage of "role diffusion," as Erikson has phrased it. It is characterized by the selection of shifting, fleeting roles, and of variable ideas, ideals, and values. At one moment an adolescent is dedicated to high idealism and resolute standards; at another moment he has seemingly abandoned both. Through normal impulses he goes forward and backward, now obnoxious or even destructive in his independence and heedlessness, now unashamedly immature, dependent, and babylike.

SUMMARY

What I have proposed here is a theoretical approach to more meaningful diagnoses of patients in the personality developmental ages. Diagnoses made in reference to maturation, maturation arrest, or regression in respect to age-expected task solution should lead to better prognosis.

Any static system of nosological nomenclature is inadequate, because no terms in themselves can picture the total personality development of the child, or can give evidence of the child's ego strengths, or can supply a hint as to the future in the great majority of behavioral disabilities. It is precisely in those cases where we can point rather accurately to the age, and to the attendant task failures of that age, that we are able to diagnose autism, phobia, obsessive-compulsive states, and so forth. Without this chronological insight, other syndromes are difficult or impossible to classify.

The great difficulty in diagnosing youthful disabilities is that in child psychiatry we are dealing with an organism while it is in the process of developing; it is developing or not developing directly in proportion to success or failure in past development, in reaction to the solutions of previous developmental tasks. To expect that we can arrive at discrete, distinct, noncomplicated states or disease entities is quite unrealistic.

It seems to me that in child psychiatry two diagnostic evaluations must be made, in relation to chronological age and in relation to personality development age. First, the diagnostic evaluation must be related cross-sectionally to the task failure in respect to the behavioral disability of the development moment or in reference to the immediate past. Although this diagnostic evaluation is usually made first, and can therefore be termed the "primary evaluation," it is really made in reference to a secondary disability or series of disabilities. Second, the diagnostic evaluation must be related to the basic developmental fault inculcated in infancy or the preschool years, and usually resulting in a series of developmental faults. Though primary and basic in respect to psychodynamic understanding of the case, this evaluation is termed the necessary "secondary diagnosis."

When both the primary and secondary evaluations or age-level diagnoses have been made (including the designation of what tasks the child has solved successfully for his present age level), then and only then can a prognosis be cited with any degree of accuracy. The best type and the proper degree of treatment can then be offered with the gratest chance of establishing the needed maturation of the moment and of ensuring proper maturation in the future.

REFERENCE

1. GARDNER, GEORGE E. Psychiatric problems of adolescence, *in* American handbook of psychiatry, ed. Silvano Arieti. New York, Basic Books, 1959. Vol. I, pp. 870–892.